LIVES WELL LIVED

R M RAGMAN

Table of Contents

Introduction

Why this book?

When someone starts to write, there must be a purpose. This writer wanted to deliver a story full of positivity. His focus would be the interaction between people. The book might give the reader a chance to think about some positive thoughts, possibly discuss these thoughts with others, and/or implement some of these thoughts into their personal lives.

The author decided on a 19th century starting point. Life might have been somewhat simpler in rural America in those days. There are no dates or other historical information mentioned in the book. They weren't necessary to the story being told. The focus of the book involves three themes: life lessons, love story, and Christian living. The life lessons and love story are intermingled throughout most of the story. Christian living seems to fit perfectly with the design of the book.

The life lessons in the book promote positivity. If individuals are focused on positive interactions with others, especially the young, great things will follow. In time, positivity might even dominate the interaction in an extended family and maybe beyond. If so, maybe negativity is put on a "back burner". I hope that this burner is buried way in the back and magically burns itself out to a large degree.

Some people grow up without learning what positivity does for others. A kind word, a smile, a compliment, a helping hand, or just being friendly are examples of being positive that promote pleasantness. These things make the world a better place in the author's opinion. Being polite and respectful are key ingredients in making any social interaction more enjoyable. When smiles, laughter, compliments, and kindness are "stirred" into the conversation, everybody benefits. There are too many words in print or floating in the air for all to hear that are not respectful, polite, or, you might add, helpful. Hence, the need for a book that is positive in nature.

The author wishes that some of the lessons in this book had been taught to him as a teenager. He would have enjoyed knowing about the power of a smile, the motivating effect of a compliment, and the mood changing ability of kind words or a helping hand.

To those kind and supportive people who smile and compliment often, you make the world a better place. Thank you with the utmost respect and admiration for what you do.

Chapter 1

Nate's Big Question

The JT Ranch was a well-run, well maintained, and highly successful endeavor that started as a small family operation. The ranch was a result of a number of life-changing events that took place over time; some of which make for an interesting story. The story begins some 50 years earlier.

"Pa," said his 11 year old son, Nate (short for Nathaniel), "you've always told me the Lord likes it when I make good use of my time, right? Well Pa, I am wasting my time going to school. I have done all the lessons and completed every book. Miss Bridgeman wants me to help the other students. I know that makes sense, but I just cannot. I want to help Dr. and Mrs. Smith. I like animals, especially horses, and I am good at working in the garden. Dr. Smith says his wife is a genius with the garden. Pa, I could learn so much. They said it would be okay if you and mom approve."

Nate's father had never heard so many words spoken by his son. As he glanced over at his son, he was not completely surprised to see that Nate was reading from a letter that he had written. Nate was not a talker. He was thoughtful, very smart, an extremely good worker for his age, and a little awkward around people. Nate's parents had talked to him about being more social, but Nate, always polite, replied that he tries, but it just does not work. This was hard for the Johnsons to understand as Pa was a minister and his mother was a schoolteacher before getting married.

"We'll talk to Miss Bridgeman and the Smiths," said Pa. "I can't promise anything. This is a big decision. Your mother and I will weigh the facts and decide what's best for you."

He was tempted to say no right now but did not want to disregard all of Nate's work in preparing his speech. School was important; there was much to learn besides the academic lessons. He would talk to his wife about it. This was Mary's area of expertise as she had taught school for 4 years and was highly acclaimed. These words from Nate caught Mr. Johnson by surprise, and, for once, he didn't know what to say. What his son said made sense. The vet and his wife were wonderful people. They had taken quite a liking to Nate. Mr. Johnson felt the Smiths would be skilled teachers. He also knew they could use Nate's energy around their house to do chores. Several people had mentioned to the minister that Mrs. Smith didn't seem to have the energy she once had.

Mr. Johnson had seen Nate's energy the last couple of years. Nate, the oldest of three children, did most of the gardening, helped with the animals, and assisted his dad on many projects around the property. Nate even made several birdhouses all by himself. They were quite good. Nate gave them to his dad to sell as Mr. Johnson supplemented his income by selling items made of wood. The only thing Nate wanted in return was a journal as his was completely full. Nate liked to write down the things he learned.

Nate seemed to feel great pleasure from work. Maybe this was because he didn't have to talk. He didn't really have any friends. His dad had never seen him talk to a girl. At town socials, Nate was always doing one of three things: eating with Dr. and Mrs. Smith, watching the other kids play, or tending to the horses and buggies. It concerned the Johnsons that their son didn't join in, but God works in mysterious ways. Most important was the fact that Nate didn't seem unhappy. He didn't laugh like other kids, play like other kids, and seemed happiest when working, unlike most other kids. Mr. Johnson also noticed that Nate smiled most often when he was working. He also smiled quite a bit when he was with the Smiths.

The Johnsons were both extremely personable. They were also very curious about the interest the Smiths were showing in their oldest child. There was no doubt that the Smiths were the most well liked couple in town, and the Johnsons were 99% sure, everything was fine. Why were the Smiths so interested in their son when these two pillars of the community, who knew everyone, could have their pick of friends or activities? They discreetly asked around. Mary did most of the inquiries, as she was a natural. The findings concurred with what the Johnsons already knew. The Smiths were great!

The Smiths were a positive and supportive force to everyone in town, especially towards children. A couple of the older townsfolk independently mentioned that the Smiths had seen a need and jumped in to help and support. There was absolutely no doubt that the Smiths made town gatherings a pleasant experience for Nate. Mr. Johnson had once overheard Dr. Smith introduce Nate to a new couple in town. The friendly doctor mentioned to the couple that they were always so happy when Nate would join them for a visit at these town gatherings. Mary also found out that a younger Thomas and Marjorie couldn't have children. Her eyes watered up when she told her husband.

The Johnsons did talk to the parties involved. Mr. Johnson talked to Miss Bridgeman the next day. The teacher stated that Nate was correct when he said he had done all the lessons. She explained, "Nate has passed his eighth grade testing with near-perfect scores. He has read my library of books up through the ninth grade and displayed complete knowledge on each one with his written reports. I've taught school for ten years at two different schools, and Nate is as quick and avid a learner as I've ever had." She said that she didn't exactly know what a genius was, but the teacher imagined Nate was as close to one as she had ever seen. He really has completed his schooling even though he is only in the fifth grade. She only wanted him to help the other students in order to develop his social skills. She was fully aware that it could be difficult for him. That's why she told Nate to think it over and talk to his parents. The decision would be entirely up to Nate's parents. Aha, thought Mr. Johnson, that's the reason for the note.

Mr. Johnson relayed all the information to his wife after dinner that night. She listened, smiled, and touched his arm as she thanked him for being so thorough. Now it was her turn to speak her mind and for her husband to listen. She was ready and knew her husband was open-minded and fair to judge. She explained, "It is critically important to ME that Nate be put in a positive situation. This is instrumental in our son's journey to manhood. A step in the wrong direction at this time might be somewhat damaging. Nate is still fragile. As he grows older, he might be able to handle a setback but not now. Continuing in school might be negative in a number of ways. Teaching other students might not work out at all. Nate needs to take baby steps. You know I don't like that 'sink or swim' mentality. I have gotten Nate to hug me back a little. It is much better than it used to be. The Smiths know Nate and can deliver the correct methods to help our son. Mrs. Smith is the most personable individual I have ever met. Her charisma fills a room. Everyone loves her; I wouldn't be surprised if Nate did too. I am a little jealous, but I believe she could do wonders for Nate. It's hard for me to say this without crying, but I'm willing to share my son with Marjorie."

Jeremy spoke in response, "Mary, you are so well thought out, and your words are absolutely correct. Our children are so lucky to have you. I wouldn't be the minister or man that I am without you. I am lucky and blessed to have God guiding me and you helping me. I truly mean this. I wasn't sure which direction to go, but your explanation, knowledge, and experience in this matter have provided the perfect path for our son. I am in perfect agreement with you." With those words he stood up, pulled her up, kissed her, and said, "Thank you and I love you."

The next day was Friday. Mrs. Johnson walked Nate to school as she did from time to time. After dropping him off, she stopped by the Smiths' house. They were both in the garden. "Hi Marjorie, Thomas," said Mrs. Johnson as she walked up, "How are you two? You're keeping the weeds down I see."

Dr. Smith had seen Mary walk up. He had been on his knees tending to a large tomato plant. As she arrived, he stood up, faced their guest with that wonderful smile of his on display, and said, "We're just great. We love working in the garden."

"Thomas has told all the weeds to go to your garden. He said the soil is so much better there," said a smiling Mrs. Smith.

Mary countered, "Thank you so very much, Thomas. The children do enjoy them. They sometimes argue over who gets to 'play' with them. We will send the bugs over here as you have such wonderfully green leaves. How do you do it?"

Thomas spoke, "Marjorie sings and talks to the plants. She sings when they are doing well and can lecture them rather sternly if needed. It does wonders." Mrs. Johnson thanked the Smiths for the tips. She always enjoyed the Smiths. They could teach Nate SO MUCH.

Marjorie asked, "Would you like a dozen carrots? We have so many; Thomas could count them as he is better at math." She smiled again.

"I could count all the way to sixteen if you'd like," laughed Thomas.

The humor was not lost. Mary understood it, appreciated it, and knew Nate would grow to love it. Smiles and laughs are so important to a childlike Nate. He knows that he belongs when he hears laughter and sees smiles. These two wonderful people had many smiles and so much more to give.

Mary responded with a smile of her own and said, "You two make a great team. One picks and the other counts. We'll have to invite you over for the apple harvest."

"Count us in," said Mr. Smith.

"You're so punny," said Marjorie.

Mary said, "You are funny, both of you. Thank you for the offer, but we have so many carrots ourselves. It has been a great year for carrots. I don't want to keep you. I just hope the bugs won't foil your toil in the soil." The Smiths laughed, but Mary went on, "Were you serious about Nate coming over here to learn and work?"

Marjorie exclaimed, "We would absolutely love it! Nate would be such a big help, which we could use, and we have a substantial library. Thomas could teach him some animal things, and I would chip in where I could. Thomas and I agree 100%. We would keep everything flexible, depending on your family needs. As Thomas would say, 'Count us in."

Mary thanked them for being so kind. She had tears in her eyes. She asked, "Can we come by this afternoon or sometime this weekend to discuss what's going to happen? We want you to know that the hours, days, and duration are completely your call."

Mrs. Smith spoke, "Thomas has a date with a mare at noon today. They are going to spend some time together, and when they are done, there will, hopefully, be a new member to our community. Can we meet at church on Sunday, right after the thoughtful sermon your husband always delivers? We are so lucky to have such a wonderful minister. Would that be OK?"

Mary answered, "Sounds great. I'll talk to Miss Bridgeman about Sunday after church at the church." Mary noticed that for a brief second Marjorie's smile left her face, but it came back quickly as Thomas, who had seen the same thing, took her hand. Mary knew what was coming next.

Thomas spoke, "Count us in." He smiled; Mary smiled right back. His smile, like Marjorie's, was contagious. He finished, "Sorry, I couldn't help myself."

Mary walked back to school just before it was time to dismiss the children. She had been curious about Marjorie's smile disappearance all day, but the former teacher told herself that she was making a mountain out of a molehill. She would inform Miss Bridgeman of the meeting right after church on Sunday. It wouldn't take long; Nate could wait by the swings.

As school was dismissed, Mary walked over to Miss Bridgeman and said, "Good day,

Miss Bridgeman. I hope your day went well."

"Busy, busy, busy," said the teacher.

Mrs. Johnson started out, "We're sorry to say that Nate will be leaving school after today. We would like to thank you for all the teaching you provided for our son, but we are enrolling him in the Smith Veterinary Clinic and Gardening Seminar. You have been a wonderful teacher. We know that Nate might have really been a benefit to the other students, but we feel this is a better fit. Would you like to come to a meeting after church to discuss Nate's future?"

Miss Bridgeman's answer spoke volumes about how she felt about Nate's move, "Mrs. Johnson, the choice was yours. You have made it. I have no input once he leaves this classroom. Tell Nate good luck; he was a very fine student. Good day to you, Mrs.

Johnson."

As Mary walked away after she wished Miss Bridgeman a good weekend, she thought Miss Bridgeman's response to Nate's leaving school provided much insight into Marjorie's reaction. Maybe Marjorie had also seen that attitude from Miss Bridgeman. This would explain the change in facial expression along with Thomas taking hold of her hand.

On Sunday, the meeting took place inside the church right after the congregation left. Minister Johnson was thanking people outside the church for coming and visiting with those who lingered behind. He always felt there might be a need that had to be addressed then or in the very near future. He was there for his congregation and didn't take the work lightly. Mary could get the meeting started. She had thought out a time frame that she believed would give the family some time with Nate in the morning. She would pack Nate a lunch, and he would head off to the Smiths' house shortly before 10:00 a.m... His departure back home would be flexible, but the plan would generally entail Nate being sent on his way around 3:30 p.m. The Smiths would tell Nate each day when they needed him for the near future.

There would be many variables in the design for Nate to help the Smiths. The lessons would be integrated into the equation. The Smiths would be completely in charge of the teaching. The key to this arrangement working well would be its flexibility. Mary knew the Smiths would be easy to work with, as it was their nature. By the time Jeremy arrived on the scene, the meeting was over.

Chapter 2
the Smiths

Dr. Smith and his wife were wonderful people. They had met in college where she was a literature major, and Thomas was in veterinary medicine. It was love at first sight for Thomas. He saw her talking with some friends. The moment Marjorie came into view Thomas felt a sensation. It was something that he had never felt before. He had looked at many girls before, but this was different. He noticed that the group was signing up for a school play. He had very little interest in acting, but he signed up anyway. It would give him a chance to talk to a young woman who had his heart all-aflutter. Thomas was very good at charming people. He had a quick smile and a very good sense of humor. When he approached Marjorie, his brain and mouth didn't work together. He stumbled badly with everything. He apologized and explained that he had never in his life ever talked to someone as beautiful as Marjorie. He quickly walked away.

In the second encounter between the college seniors, Thomas was back to his normal self. He smiled, laughed at himself, and explained why he had been so nervous. He had wanted to ask Marjorie to go to a school musical on Saturday afternoon. Marjorie was impressed with his contagious smile. You couldn't help smiling when he smiled. She really liked that. He was also quite good looking. She said yes to the musical. They met outside the auditorium. They had a great time being together. The couple smiled and laughed often, and several times during the performance, Thomas held her hand. She really liked that. After such an enjoyable time, Thomas asked Marjorie out on a real date for next Saturday.

After what happened on their first real date, Marjorie knew this was the man she would marry. They were having some dinner at a restaurant when Thomas saw a man staring into the eatery from outside. Thomas excused himself, went outside, and the next thing you know, the man was sitting at the table. Thomas introduced him; he appeared to be down on his luck. Thomas asked him many questions over the next thirty minutes as all the food was consumed. Thomas finished the conversation by telling Bill to come to the front of the college at 9:30 sharp the next morning. Bill agreed, shook Thomas' hand, thanked him for being so kind, and said that he would see Thomas tomorrow. After Bill left, Thomas took Marjorie's hands and said, "I'm so sorry about ruining our date, but I couldn't help myself. Bill looked so hungry and sad. I had to help." Marjorie leaned over the table and gave Thomas a long kiss.

They were married about six months later. They lived with Thomas' parents. Thomas' dad was a local vet who also taught at the college. After Thomas graduated, he joined his father's practice. Marjorie had quit school after she and Thomas were married. She knew what she wanted. She would support Thomas and his career, run the household, and take care and nurture the children. It was important to know as much as possible about the practice as she wanted to lighten Thomas' load of responsibilities.

Things were great for a couple of years, but there was mounting pressure to have children. It came mostly from friends and relatives. Bart and "Millie" were great either way. They loved their only child and adored Marjorie. They explained to the newlyweds that it hadn't been easy for them to get pregnant either. They mentioned that people don't mean to be nosy. It is just a topic of conversation that is always brought up with newlyweds. It will die down. Ours did after several years. The young married couple also, over time, started to get a feeling that maybe it was time to begin a plan to be on their own. They truly valued their alone time.

In the third year of working with his dad in the practice, Thomas and Marjorie decided it was time to branch out on their own. There was a need for a vet many miles to the west in a small but growing town. Thomas had been able to save a rather large portion of his pay from the practice, and Marjorie came from money although you would never know it. She never mentioned it to anyone. Thomas was the only one who knew. They certainly had enough startup money. It was a sad goodbye because the opportunity was a couple of hundred miles away.

Thomas and Marjorie loved their new town. The people were friendly and thankful for the Smiths' arrival. They kept busy making acquaintances in town and beyond. It didn't take long for the Smiths to make friends. They stayed in the local hotel for a short time as Thomas and a few hired workers built the barn and office for Dr. Smith's practice. The project took about a week and a half. Thomas and Marjorie moved into it as a temporary residence. Marjorie had ordered more supplies during the barn building, and Dr. Smith was ready to see "patients" right after the move to their new quarters.

The house was going to be Marjorie's job. Thomas told her that she had more style and taste in her pinky finger than he had in his whole body. All decisions from the materials, design, and the actual building were hers to make. She knew what she wanted along with the knowledge of what Thomas liked. It was to be built with good workmanship using fine materials, not too fancy but nice. She explained to Thomas that this was going to be our "castle" for many years. They were both very excited about their own place.

Marjorie hired a talented builder named Jake Collins who, like them, had traveled west to make a name for himself. He had been trained by his highly skilled dad as a finish carpenter. Marjorie and Jake met and came up with a design. In ten weeks, Jake and his two hired hands completed the house. Marjorie handled the whole production while paying Jake and the workers as the house progressed. She paid Jake and his crew well but asked them not to discuss the amount. She explained to them that it was private business and would like to keep it that way.

Courier from a bank had delivered all the money for materials and wages paid by Marjorie to Jake forty miles away. Marjorie did not want people to know of her wealth. Of course, there would be some talk, but no one would know for sure. She knew gossip was a favorite hobby of many small town locals. Marjorie knew how gossip worked and learned long ago that it generally died away without some facts to support it. She did not want people to like her for her money or to treat her special because of her wealth. What she really would enjoy was for people to like her for her good deeds and positive interactions with all the residents of the town.

Marjorie didn't want Thomas to worry about the new house, as he was busy working and meeting the town folks. Of course, he peeped in after work and loved what he saw. He told his wife often that she was very amazing. This made her so happy because she wanted the house to be special for her Thomas. It was.

The design and workmanship were splendid. Jake had a real knack for creativity and the skills to make it become a reality. Thomas knew some about woodworking and wished he could watch Jake work, but he didn't know him well enough to ask. Thomas couldn't stop praising the builders and Marjorie. Truth be told, any house would have been fine as long as it had Marjorie in it. She brightened every day, and now this house was to be their sanctuary. It was to be a place where they would share so much.

In four months, the Smiths had settled in and were doing very well. Marjorie was helping in the practice, volunteering at the small local church, and planning to start a small library in an old abandoned building. She was also preparing the soil for next year's garden. The Smiths had also planted two apple trees. Thomas used to kid, "I hope an apple a day won't keep the doctor away." He always hugged M while he was saying it, and she always kissed him after he finished. It never got old. That is how much in love they were.

Thomas still enjoyed calling Marjorie M in private. It was such a special word for both of them. Marjorie loved it when he called her M. There was so much love attached to the nickname. M had, of course, asked Thomas if she could give him a nickname. He responded, "When you touch my hand, face, or arm and say Thomas, it melts my heart. It never gets old, and I love it more and more. Please just continue that for," he paused, "forever and a day." She responded with the taking of his hand along with the words that it would be her pleasure. M then gave Thomas a big hug and kiss.

After nine years, the Smiths were pillars of the community. The town had tripled in size, and there were many town meetings to discuss improvements to accommodate all the new members of town. The Smiths were a positive force in supporting town activities. Not only did they volunteer, they contributed monetarily without anyone knowing, with the exception of the mayor. Even he wasn't sure how much they gave.

Marjorie had a great way of getting things done without expounding on who did this or gave this amount. She was always the representative at town gatherings after the mayor spoke. She always thanked the town with words like, "So many gave for the cost of materials that it just warms my heart to be here in such a fine and caring town". Of course, the town folks loved these words because Marjorie spoke from her heart. The people saw this and always responded. She would spend more time thanking the volunteers. She would mention specific projects that were handled by the town volunteers. Marjorie explained how so very special this was because the town had built it.

She never mentioned people's names. In doing this, she felt that everybody could feel appreciated for what they personally did, no matter how big or small. This was important to Marjorie because she knew that people gave what they could. Some could do more, but the ones who couldn't give much should not be slighted in any way. The town residents loved Marjorie's words, her thoughts, and her kindness for all. Marjorie would have been mayor by unanimous decree if she had been a man. She knew this and understood that this was the way of the world. She also knew these people were her extended family, and she would never let them down.

The Smiths loved volunteering. The couple was so happy being together as a team and making everybody laugh as they all worked together. Thomas and Marjorie always did as much work or more than the other volunteers did. It was just their way; they led by example. Many of the local folks looked to the Smiths as examples of lives well lived.

Of course, it didn't come as any surprise that when the new larger church and school were to be the next town project, the Smiths were there to assist. Jake Collins and his crew would be the builders for much of the church and would be compensated. Most of the town people would volunteer, when and wherever possible. Marjorie would lead the committee to raise the money. The most popular person in town insisted the work be started before the funds were raised. The initial fundraiser did well, and she felt that more funds would be easily gathered.

The mayor agreed after Marjorie talked to him, and the work by the hired personnel and volunteers eagerly began. The money did flow in; the new church and school were soon finished. They were beautiful. There was even a small cottage for the schoolteacher very near the school and a nice home about a half mile out of town for the minister.

Marjorie was not involved in the choosing of a new minister and teacher. She decided it was important to tastefully step aside and let the rest of the town committee make the choice. The previous teacher was well liked by the parents and excellent with the children. Unfortunately, for the town, but great for the young teacher, she got married and was moving to a different town. Typical of the people in the town, they gave her a huge wedding shower and a wonderful send-off with many fine gifts. Of course, Marjorie was the organizer of the event.

The pastor was a local farmer; he and the town decided it was time for a full-time minister. After some contacts and letter writing, the committee made their choices. Miss Bridgeman was to be the new teacher, and Mr. and Mrs. Johnson would be moving into the minister's house, along with their two-year-old son, Nathanial.

Chapter 3

Nate's Growth

Over the next number of years, Nate worked with the Smiths, his dad, and the town blacksmith. He learned so much that he filled eight journals. The journals were sophisticated and full of great information and insight. This opinion came from Nate's father, who had read each one carefully and truly believed they were publishable.

Nate was thriving in so many ways. It appeared that Nate quitting school had been the right decision in his quest to reach manhood. He had gained a confidence that allowed him to speak more openly about any topic he might be working on. When people asked a question, he would give them a relatively complete answer, and sometimes he might even throw in a smile or laugh. He had his own ideas that he would share with those close to him. His work was deliberate and refined, much appreciated by everyone. He wasn't your normal apprentice; he was so much more.

The Johnsons also saw a rather large change in Nate's personality. He showed more emotion. This was something he rarely did as a younger boy. He regularly hugged his mother with him initiating the act. He also hugged his brother and sister. When he shook his dad's hand, Nate would take his dad's hand with both of his as he smiled with some emotion. Occasionally, Mr. Johnson had seen Dr. Smith and Nate shake hands in a similar fashion. How could he be jealous of a man who had taught his son so much? He couldn't. Mary felt the same about Marjorie. Mrs. Johnson had some input about Nate's "schooling" when she and Marjorie would talk, but there was no doubt who was teaching their son about the social and emotional realm of life. Mary would often cry tears of joy when talking to Jeremy about their son's growth. Both the Johnsons truly believed divine intervention had brought the Smiths into Nate's life.

Nate still did not have any real friends. It didn't bother him in the least. He had five adults who he was very close with. His interaction with them took up most of his time. He did know other people and conversed much more than in the past. He was always polite and pleasant. The Johnsons liked his progress. Nate did seem to enjoy his brother and sister. They would ask him questions. He always gave them an answer with a complete explanation if necessary. The back and forth included smiles and touches on the shoulder and an occasional laugh aloud. It was wonderful to see. Nate always listened intently to his siblings and commented on their words. He showed them a kindness the Johnsons hadn't seen when he was younger.

Nate had always made things for people or helped someone in need. This showed the true nature of his character and the kindness within. These qualities helped create a bond between the three children that was quite special. Their parents couldn't have been prouder of the love that had developed between the three siblings. One Sunday after dinner as Nate was getting ready to go home (he had moved to a small cabin behind the Smiths when he was eighteen), he gave out three big hugs and a great big handshake to his father. Mary never got tired of this. Nate went to the other room and came back with two wrapped presents for his brother and sister. Inside were two of the finest plagues Mr. Johnson had ever seen. They were a combination of wrought iron and wood, fine hardwood. Engraved rather exquisitely by hand were the words:

"God and I will always look over you"

Your brother Nate

There wasn't a dry eye in the house. For the first time since Nate started work with the Smiths, Mary wished they could have been here to witness this.

The Smiths paid Nate a salary for his work. At first, it wasn't very much, a little more than age appropriate. By the age of sixteen, Nate was more like a hired hand in terms of work. He could handle the garden completely, do things for Dr. Smith independently, or cook a meal if needed. Accordingly, the Smiths increased Nate's wages. At no time was there talk about the strong bond that had developed between the three. The Smiths thought it would be inappropriate to discuss such a topic with Nate. They did not want to interfere with the Johnson family dynamics. Their purpose was to benefit Nate, but they both knew it was more than that. Nate felt the same feeling towards the Smiths. He really enjoyed the adults in his life, but the feelings he had for the Smiths were the strongest emotions that he had ever experienced. He felt very lucky and blessed but wasn't ready to talk about it. It was a little confusing.

There were a number of times when Dr. Smith needed some work done at the local blacksmith shop. At the age of fifteen, Nate started watching the local blacksmith, a big Negro man named Jack Brown. Jack had come to town several years ago to help the existing blacksmith who had hurt his back. The back never got better, so Jack took over the business. He always paid the owner a salary until he died. Jack Brown was a good man, funny and kind, who just happened to have the best singing voice in church. He also knew his craft extremely well. Dr. Smith said that Jack could pound iron better than anyone he had ever seen.

Mr. Brown, that is what Nate called him, started kidding Nate when he came by that Nate should start working with him to put some muscles "on demb bones". In a short time, Nate was working with Mr. Brown. Jack was patient, kind, and a great teacher. Nate loved the work and really appreciated Mr. Brown. By the time he was nearing eighteen, the muscles were there, along with a significant amount of skill. His mother even commented on his muscles and physique. Two days later Marjorie made the same comments and added that Nate had become a handsome young man. Nate really enjoyed the compliments. Once again, on both occasions, he was able to experience the joy of receiving compliments.

Nate and his dad even added wrought iron to some of their designs. It added another dimension and made these projects quite special. Some were taken by a local vendor to the nearest big town to sell. They normally always sold well. Jack Brown and Nate's dad both insisted that Nate be paid for his work. Nate refused, but the two adults explained that since Nate was doing a man's job with great skill, he should be paid. Mr. Brown, in his deep smooth voice, calmly said, "Nate, you are a young man now. Men get paid for their work." As Jack spoke these words, Nate's father was smiling and nodding his head. Jeremy seemed to be so proud.

All Nate could say was, "Okay", but inside he was bursting with emotion. These two amazing men just agreed that he was a young man, and his work was great. These compliments were powerful. Nate would savor them for quite some time. He also knew that these were the types of compliments he would love handing out.

On most Saturdays and Sundays after Nate turned eighteen and was living in his own place, he worked and visited with his family. He still really liked working with his dad on projects. They discussed designs, materials, and different aspects of the work. What Nate really enjoyed was the fact that his dad treated him as an equal. Nate knew his dad still had many things he could teach his son but chose to be equal partners. His dad, already knowing the answer, might ask Nate questions about what type of wood grain to expose. He would ask subtle design questions that made Nate stop and think out an answer, all with the intention of enhancing his son's skills. This was how thoughtful Jeremy was, and it was a style of teaching a lesson that Nate never forgot. Ask pointed questions or guide the learner to the desired answer, with the student doing the thinking and discovering the best solution on their own. Whenever he used it later in his life, he thought of his dad.

As the family did their chores for the day, Nate jumped right in and helped everybody. He especially loved working with his brother and sister. Doris was thirteen and was in charge of the garden. Andy, age eight, would assist his sister, making sure to do as she said. It was to be a team effort with equal amounts of work, but every team needs a captain. Doris was the captain of the garden. Andy was the captain of the animals with the same rules as the garden but with him being the boss. Nate loved the setup and knew exactly who orchestrated the design. Both children got to lead, follow, work, and learn to be fair. They had to talk things out and organize. It was a perfect teaching moment designed by a perfect teacher. Gosh, mom was smart. Another lesson learned that Nate never forgot.

As Jeremy would go over his sermon for the next day, the four others would fix dinner. Mrs. Johnson designed it, so everyone would contribute to the preparation. She made it special. Everybody laughed, sometimes to tears. She sometimes talked the children into playing the "thank you and you're welcome game". Andy's job was to keep track of the score. He felt important doing the job. Mom always won and always said that it was because she was older and had more practice saying these wonderful words. Another lesson – amazing

Sundays were fun because the family went to church together. Dad was in front with the rest of the family in the front row. As Nate grew older, he realized how skillful of a speaker his dad was, personable, knowledgeable, and very professional...

The Smiths and Johnsons started getting together occasionally for dinner on Saturdays. It was always a good time with lots of conversation and stories. The number of smiles and laughs filled the house. Mary agreed to the meals before she talked to her husband about it. Marjorie brought up the topic one afternoon as Mary, who had gone into town, dropped by to walk home with Nate.

Mary did not often make a family decision without first discussing it with Jeremy, but her gut was screaming to say yes to this incredible woman now. Immediately after being asked to share some meals, she did say yes to Marjorie about the meals. The response from Mrs. Smith was so warm. She hugged Mary and exclaimed, "These meals are going to be so much fun. Thomas and I will look forward to these occasions." Mary's gut was right virtually all the time and judging from Marjorie's facial expression, the gut didn't fail Mary this time either.

Mary did talk to Jeremy a short time later explaining that Marjorie mentioned sharing some meals together. She explained that Marjorie caught her off guard somewhat, but she could not say no. Jeremy chimed in, "You were absolutely correct to say yes."

Mary continued, "Marjorie asked what we normally have for dinner on Saturdays. After I explained one of our most typical meals, she said that they love that meal and eat it quite often. She asked if I would fix that when they came over." Mary added that Marjorie said these dinners were going to be so much fun, and the Smiths will love being part of the Johnson clan. Marjorie was smiling the whole time as she spoke. Mary finished speaking by telling Jeremy, "Marjorie touched my shoulder during the last sentence. That kind of melted my heart."

Jeremy spoke, "I think the Smiths are looking for something more than friendship. They have many, many friends, but my understanding is that they don't have any family."

Mary quickly added, "They do now."

Mary did not tell Jeremy that they would be having chicken casserole and salad upon arriving at the Smiths' abode. Marjorie had explained they usually have an abundance of chicken and, thanks to Nate, plenty of salad. Jeremy loved a chicken casserole and a fresh salad. The Johnson didn't eat much chicken because they used the chickens for eggs. Mary had heard that Marjorie was a wonderful cook. Jeremy would be so pleased and surprised. His praise and thankfulness would make Marjorie's day.

Mary also realized that Marjorie did not want the meals to be a competition between the two cooks. She purposely arranged what meals were to be eaten. Marjorie likely figured out that as smart as Mary was, she probably already deduced that the Smiths had money. Mary did know because Nate had informed his mother that sometimes Thomas was paid in chicken. There were other times when he wasn't paid at all. Dr. Smith always said to the client, "Don't worry, you can pay me later by doing me a favor." Nate said this payback very seldom happened, but Dr. Smith never stopped seeing the customer. Mary had also heard from time to time that some people did not know where all the money came from to build the church along with the two additional homes. Most of these folks suspected the Smiths contributed the money. There was no proof. The Smiths sure weren't talking, but some knew. Marjorie had planned the dinners so there was no pressure to keep up with the Smiths. It was going to be just the two families having a good time and sharing some tasty food. So thoughtful — so wonderful.

After the first meal, the Johnsons, especially Mary, thoroughly enjoyed the Smiths. Thomas and Marjorie praised the cook, interacted with the children, smiled often, and made everyone laugh. Marjorie spent most of the time before and after dinner talking to Doris and Andy. They showed her the garden and all the animals. They talked constantly, probably, because Marjorie praised their wonderful work. Her warm smiles lit up their faces; they loved it. Thomas traveled right out to the woodworking room with Nate and Jeremy. He had asked if he could see the place where they performed their magic. He explained that he was a big fan of their work. It didn't take long after a short conversation that Jeremy had Thomas involved in the project. He really enjoyed working with his hands. When he left, he thanked the Johnsons for their kindness. They, in turn, thanked him for his fine help. They all agreed to do it again. Once again, Mary was so impressed with Marjorie. She just seemed to have an ability to make people feel good. Over the years, Mary grew more and more enamored with this charming woman. She was so very special. In time the meals became a regular event. Eventually, on two days a month and every holiday, the Johnsons and Smiths shared a meal. The two families had become one.

Chapter 4
Marjorie

Marjorie was much like her mother. People said they were like twins at different ages. Pictures show this to be true. They had very similar mannerisms, smiles, and laughs. Marjorie was a bright student just as her mom had been. As Marjorie got older, she learned so much by watching her mother interact with others. There were also many oral lessons that were replicated in order that Marjorie not forget. An example of one would explain these life lessons. It happened at a restaurant, and the lesson involved saying nice things to people by using their name or emphasizing positive words if you didn't know their name. Abigail told Marjorie that people love to be complimented. It definitely builds their self-worth, improves their confidence, changes their mood in a positive way, and usually brightens their day.

"Watch our waiter after I talk to him," Mom said. She explained that he hasn't smiled since we sat down. Marjorie agreed with her mother's assessment. She watched and listened to the conversation after her mother called the waiter over to the table. "Young man, could I ask you your name please? I would like to tell the manager how knowledgeable you were when you were helping my daughter with her order. Would it be alright with you if I left a small note for your manager as a token of our appreciation?" said my mother as she smiled and touched his arm.

"My name is Dan, and it would be amazing if you left the note. Please don't feel any pressure to do so," the waiter said with a big smile on his face.

"Well, thank you, Dan, for making our lunch so pleasant," my smiling mom said. She continued after he left, "Watch him as we eat our meal. Be discreet, no eye contact. See how much he smiles and how his demeanor has changed," said the smartest woman in the room. Mom was correct. He was much more pleasant, smiled several times, and had more bounce in his step. Mom then said this works even well when you know the person. It works with your father more often than not, and you know how difficult it can be to change his mind.

Marjorie had indeed noticed how her mom interacted with Daddy. She smiled, complimented him, and said other things to inspire him. These things had to be used, Marjorie guessed, because Daddy only cared about business and money. Daddy did not smile often or tell a joke as far back as Marjorie could remember. He had a stern demeanor the majority of the time. Mom had to really convince Daddy to go on a vacation once a year. It wasn't easily accomplished, but some say Abigail had a brilliant mind and knew how to use it. It didn't hurt that she was beautiful with a warm smile to go along with it.

Vacations were the only time that Daddy did not treat his son, Henry, six years older than Marjorie, in a stern, strict manner. Mom tried to intervene, work her "magic" in a number of ways, or change the topic but nothing worked. Marjorie often heard Daddy saying things like "that's the way I was raised and look at me, rich and powerful". Marjorie heard and saw much during the years when Henry was living at home. It had a great impact on the kind of man she would marry.

Henry left home when he was eighteen, never to return. He just couldn't handle the treatment from his father any longer. One day he just packed up some of his things and left. Henry left a note explaining that he wasn't coming back, so please don't send someone for him. Mother never forgave Daddy for his harsh treatment of Henry that drove her son away. Marjorie never heard her mother complain about anything. It wasn't her nature to be negative, but one day when Marjorie walked into the study, she saw her mother holding a picture of Henry. She had been crying. Marjorie quickly went to her mother and held her for some time. Abigail simply told her caring daughter that she had a hole in her heart, and your father put it there. Marjorie continued to hold her mother while whispering things to comfort her. Abigail didn't respond in words but held her daughter very tightly. She never spoke about her husband's terrible treatment of Henry again.

Marjorie had also watched her mother interact with Daddy to do good things with his money. Daddy made it abundantly clear that it was his money. He controlled it, and there would be no handouts. He never got one and didn't intend to give one. Abigail did get her husband to give, but it always had his name attached to it. After Henry left, Daddy worked even longer hours. Marjorie saw it all. The warmth in the household was almost gone. If it hadn't been for mom and the staff, there would have been none. Daddy poisoned any room he was in. He looked much older and seemed to be drinking alcohol more often. It was terrible.

Marjorie did have some wonderful friends where she could laugh and have fun. She was already starting to use the lessons from her mother to compliment her friends, move the group in a positive direction, and help the group accomplish things it never would have without Marjorie there to lead the way. Abigail had explained to her daughter that negative conversations and gossip were not productive and generally did much more harm than good. Abigail had discussed the topic of gossip many times with her daughter. She had given many examples and explained the consequences very clearly.

The bright daughter remembered two examples that her mother taught that pointed out the character flaws in the gossipers. A pretty girl degrades another classmate's looks; she is hoping to boost herself and bring attention to her looks. SO WRONG Mother mentioned, "This girl may be pretty on the outside but, excuse my words, is ugly on the inside." A strong boy doing the same type of thing to other weaker boys shows a definite weakness of character. Marjorie never forgot these two examples, along with her mother's thoughts that every person should be treated with respect and kindness. This was why Abigail did not like bragging. She thought, at times, it made others feel bad.

Marjorie had, of course, seen gossiping at school. Abigail's lessons taught that gossip, sometimes, was a form of bullying, and bullying was just plain wrong. It was unchristian and terribly hurtful. It should never be tolerated. The word bullying never left Marjorie's mind. She saw the hurt, damage, and sadness in victims at school. She had a real disdain for bullies and gossip. Whenever she could, she went out of her way to be kind to the victims of any type of abuse. Marjorie had, of course, relayed Abigail's gossip and bullying lessons to her friends. Marjorie made it abundantly clear that these actions were just plain wrong. She explained, "We are NOT that type of people. Be positive and do good deeds; that's who we are." These words would dominate Marjorie's actions for most of her adult life. Abigail would have been so proud.

Marjorie made projects fun, always making sure everyone was involved and happy. She relished the role and often talked to her mother about projects and/or her friends. Abigail took such pride in her daughter's development. Marjorie was becoming someone quite special, not just a pretty face. One example of Marjorie's projects was the talent show. The idea came to her when she was sixteen, and she continued being the leader of the project until she left for college. Before Marjorie left, she made sure the project was safe for several more years. It was very popular for all those connected to the production, and the public loved the performances. It also made quite a bit of money for local charities.

The same popularity could be said of the school bake table. A group of girls (mostly Marjorie's friends and acquaintances) established an ongoing baked goods table at school. All the proceeds went to benefit the music program at school. Marjorie even talked her daddy into paying for a new separate music room away from other classrooms. She told her friends that her mother did all of the work in convincing Daddy to finance the building. The leader of the do-good deeds group did not want any credit for the music building; it wouldn't be right. It might even be a slight to her friends. You don't need your name attached when doing good deeds.

Seeing people benefitting from your good deeds is the greatest reward a person could ask for. Marjorie had taught her friends that it was important to do good deeds, help where possible, and contribute to the town. These things show great character. Marjorie had all her friends on board with these thoughts. Abigail was given so many compliments from the mothers of Marjorie's friends. She never told her daughter a word about all these kind words. Instead, she told her daughter frequently that she was doing a wonderful job helping so many and doing such positive things. She always finished with a big long hug, along with the words, "I'm so proud of you".

Abigail valued the time she spent with her only child left at home. Marjorie felt the same way and told her mom occasionally, "I love my friends, but my mother is the most important person in the world to me. My love for her knows no bounds." This was always followed by a big hug and a few dabs of handkerchiefs to the eyes by both mother and daughter.

Marjorie would especially look forward to those special days when she and her mother would dress up and go to lunch in a nearby town. The trip would take 5-6 hours. After several trips to lunch, Daddy said at dinner one night that the lunches were a total waste of time and money. Mother explained that the food was exquisite, and she needed this time to have mother-daughter talks. Marjorie had eaten earlier at a friend's house, but she was downstairs and could hear the conversation. She was intrigued by what was going to happen next. She peeked around the corner to see and listen. Mother explained as she smiled that a daughter at a certain age needs to talk to her mother about certain female issues. These mother-daughter conversations are critical to her development.

"Don't you think that this is important stuff?" she said.

"You can't do it here," Daddy countered.

"Going to lunch makes it special, and it has to be special. One day soon Marjorie will be leaving our home. She will remember our mother-daughter talks if I make them special enough. It is something I must do for our daughter. You can't do it. I must do this; I enjoy every moment of it. It's my job." She paused and then spoke in a near whisper with eyes slightly watering, "Do you understand?"

"Yes, I understand," said Daddy. It was never brought up again. Marjorie once again witnessed her mother perform her magic, but she was troubled somewhat. It wasn't completely honest.

Years later, Marjorie would talk to a minister about convincing people into your way of thinking. It was a long conversation over dinner. The young woman had many questions. It was decided in the end that being completely honest would be best, but, occasionally, a person can convince others to do something by leaving out some pertinent facts or truths for the greater good. The minister emphasized the word occasionally again but also said he deals with this question in his ministry. The man of the church believed the times he convinced people to go in a particular direction always worked well for everybody. He smiled and said that he had someone helping him. He encouraged Marjorie to pray on such matters and follow your heart. Thinking back to that conversation between Mother and Daddy that had bothered her, Marjorie felt relieved. It was definitely for the greater good.

Occasionally, Henry would join them for lunch. He lived in a town some distance away but would make the trip. THESE DAYS WERE WAY BEYOND SPECIAL. There was so much love, smiles, hugs, laughter, and a few tears. Marjorie was only fourteen on the first lunch with Henry, but she learned so much from listening to the conversation. After that lunch, she was participating as an equal, giving and receiving in the joy of the occasion. Marjorie had never seen her mom so happy, and Henry was a completely different person. Daddy never did find out why these lunches took so long.

Of course, Mom and Henry had never stopped communicating. Abigail arranged for Henry's mail to be sent to the local library addressed to the head librarian, a very good friend of Abigail's. Abigail would send her mail through another friend's husband who owned a construction company. These two friends loved Abigail and had a rather large dislike for her husband. They were more than glad to help.

At age twenty-two, Henry sent his last letter explaining that he and his best friend were going to the gold fields. He apologized for not having lunch before he went, but he couldn't do this in person, as he couldn't bear to see the pain. Marjorie and Abigail would never hear from Henry again. Marjorie was saddened and cried some, but her friends comforted her. Abigail was devastated. She was more reserved, gone from home more, and the lunches stopped. Henry was not a topic of conversation ever. Marjorie also noticed her amazing mother's eyes were sometimes red when she came home.

Six weeks after Henry's letter, Abigail sat Marjorie down one afternoon for a little conversation. She explained that Daddy used to want to travel to famous places, dress up in expensive clothing, and wear some very fine jewelry. Abigail explained very carefully to her daughter, "This was totally unacceptable to me. It is just not who I am. To flaunt your wealth in such a manner is arrogant and has an air of superiority, in my opinion. Both of these words make my stomach upset. Don't get me wrong. It is perfectly okay for folks to do this. They have earned it and have the right to spend their money as they choose. I personally like to help others, do good deeds, and not draw attention to myself. I hope you are the same way. I repeat; I truly hope you are."

"One day you will receive some of your daddy's money. Promise me you will never flaunt your wealth. Use the money instead to help people and build things that benefit many. I am not asking you to go without. Live comfortably, enjoy nice things, but don't use all your money on yourself and your family."

Marjorie took her mother's hand and said, "I feel the same way. I have seen some rich people do as you say, and it bothered me. Your lessons for me make me more like you, and, Mom, I aspire to be you. Thank you for this lesson, and I love you more than words could say."

Mother and daughter embraced. Abigail finished the conversation by telling her daughter that they needed to get back to doing good deeds and helping others. Marjorie then knew her mom had bounced back from the pain of Henry's leaving. Another lesson taught by Mom that Marjorie never wanted to experience again.

Six months after Henry left for the gold fields, Marjorie's sister, Sarah, came home from an elite college. Daddy had insisted that Sarah attend the school in order to meet the right people and possibly the right person. Daddy was big on the right people. He never said it, but he meant the people with a prestigious family name and the connections that go along with it. Wealth had to be part of the equation, the more, the better. Daddy believed in wealth, connections, and family name in that order. He really loved money and the power it brought. Abigail had opposed the whole idea of that particular school, but Daddy won that battle.

Sarah didn't look healthy when she got home. She was always somewhat quiet but even more so now. Abigail suspected that she had been a victim at school. Such schools were notorious for their cruelty to the shy and quiet. This is what Abigail was afraid of all along. She would restart the nurturing and love that had seemed to work well before Sarah had gone away. She could only hope that a mom's care could restore her daughter back to normal.

Six months later, Sarah was much improved. Abigail felt there was still a need to build Sarah's sense of self-worth. It was damaged at school and was going to take time to mend. Sarah was nearly twenty-one now, a grown woman, and wounds don't heal as quickly as they did when she was a child.

Abigail didn't get the chance. Sarah had met a young man at the market. He paid attention to her and made her feel special. They started secretly meeting and a romance began. Abigail noticed the change in Sarah and asked her about it. Sarah explained that she had made a few new friends. Before Abigail could invite these "friends" over for an afternoon snack and visit, Sarah ran off with her new friend, Johnny, and got married.

When the couple returned with the news, Daddy was beyond furious. He threatened to have Johnny thrown in jail and have the marriage annulled, but the parents were helpless. Johnny and Sarah were adults. Abigail was saddened that her daughter had not confided in her. She knew Sarah was vulnerable, but Abigail hoped she had built Sarah's self-esteem to the extent that this situation wouldn't arise. Daddy stormed around for weeks, yelling about the scandal that Sarah caused and the embarrassment to the family. It was going to cost him a boatload of money and damage his business connections. He blamed Abigail for not raising Sarah correctly. Abigail was smart enough not to add fuel to the fire. She knew who caused the whole mess but chose to say repeatedly, "I'm sorry." She knew things could get worse. They did.

Sarah and Johnny wrote a letter to Daddy explaining how much in love they were. They apologized for the elopement, but explained they couldn't wait. Surely, he could understand. In the last part of the letter, the young couple asked for some start-up money. Johnny had a job and Sarah was going to get one, but right now, they needed money for a place to live, along with the furnishings to accompany it.

Daddy did more than just reject their request. He had his will redone, cutting the married couple off completely. Not only that, he cut off anybody in the family who gave the couple money or anything of value. He knew that Abigail would try to support her daughter. She always babied the children and gave them too much. If she went against his wishes, she would get nothing. He no longer cared about Abigail. She had crossed him too many times. HE WOULD WIN THIS BATTLE. He would show his wife who had the power and the control in the family.

Abigail did help the young married couple. What else could she do? It was her daughter. Over the years, Abigail had built up a nest egg from the household funds and dress money. She used it for different types of projects. Now Abigail used it to funnel money to Sarah. The young couple seemed to always need money, and the funds were soon gone. Abigail tried to continue to help, but she was venturing into an area that her husband was a master in. Soon he caught Abigail and the staff stealing money from the household funds. The first thing he did was fire the entire staff. Abigail tried to defend them and their innocence, but her husband would not listen. He hired a new staff that answered only to him and did his bidding. Abigail no longer had anything to do with running the household. Any money she needed would have to be requested through the head of the staff. In addition to this slap in the face, Abigail was no longer part of the will.

Throughout the years, Abigail made many dresses for Sarah and Marjorie. The sewing was always done at her best friend's house. Abigail had a real talent taught to her by her mother. The dresses were exquisite and Daddy did not hesitate to pay the price. His daughters had to look special as they traveled around town to nice places. It was good for business and caught the eye of just the right people who frequented these establishments. Daddy thought the dresses were store bought. The receipts were from a local upscale dress shop. What he didn't know was the receipts were fake, courtesy of the owner of the shop, a good friend of Abigail's. Abigail stashed the money from the dresses away to help finance her projects and other items for the children that her husband wouldn't pay for.

With all the new changes at home, there was one thing that Abigail was NOT going to do. She would not stay home. The new staff was not friendly at all. They made Abigail feel uncomfortable in her own house. To make matters even worse, she felt all of this was deliberate.

Abigail had always supplied baked goods to Marjorie's school bake table. She was a talented baker, another gift from her mother. She also sold some items at her friend's bakery. Abigail was resourceful and had added this source of revenue to her stash, but now, she would have to generate money on a weekly basis. Abigail had done many helpful things for her friends. They all wanted to pay her back. Maybe it was time to ask for help. With her friends' help, she knew she could raise the money because her two revenue sources were popular with many people.

Another reason Abigail could be a success was that she went out to work on most days. She left early and came home just before her husband. There was one thing Abigail was not going to do. She would not stop helping her daughter. She still baked for Marjorie, somewhat less, but others had stepped up their production. She made a few dollars from the bakery. Abigail had enough cash to buy material for her beautifully designed dresses. Abigail enjoyed the work. Creating something original for people to enjoy brought her great joy. She had always been a creative person.

When Abigail was first married, she cooked and sewed. Soon after her husband's business success took off, he hired a complete household staff and told Abigail to stay out of the kitchen. That is when she moved her skills outside the house. Her husband never found out about her baking and sewing because he really didn't care about women is socializing. Abigail was smart enough to ask for her husband's permission to visit outside the household. She explained that it was important for a wealthy man's wife to be seen socializing around the city. She would occasionally ask for money to go out to a fancy restaurant. Her husband always agreed to this as he thought it was smart business to have the right people see his beautiful wife, dressed exquisitely, socializing at fine establishments. What he didn't know was the fact that these amazing dresses were made by Abigail.

Those days were gone. Nowadays, Abigail didn't ask to leave the house, didn't ask to visit friends, didn't ask to socialize, and would never, repeat NEVER, ask the head of the staff for money.

Abigail and Marjorie became quite a team. Marjorie and her mother had several talks about keeping things calm at home. Marjorie was to be in charge of dealing with her daddy. She was good at it, as she had learned her mother's lessons well. Abigail was okay at offering advice and strategies. She wasn't talking to her husband. The wife knew the relationship was gone, but she stayed out of Marjorie's way as her daughter took over. Marjorie knew her mother was distressed in so many ways. When Daddy wasn't around, Marjorie hugged her mother, held her hand, said kind words to her, and comforted her. Sometimes Abigail would cry, but she was getting better.

Daddy left for work very early and came back late. Marjorie knew Daddy was pretty much hated at work. He used people to make money and didn't care if he crushed a few along the way. He was about winning, making money, and increasing his power. When Marjorie thought about such things, it brought back her mother's lesson on being self-centered. The lesson was simple; a person who focuses on himself or herself often becomes selfish. Selfishness can sometimes lead to being overly competitive or possibly greedy. Both of these things are NOT GOOD. Abigail asked her daughter to please focus on others; be kind and do good things. Be as positive as possible in all your dealings with others.

Marjorie did notice that on more than one occasion, Daddy smelled of alcohol when he left for work in the morning. He was missing more and more family dinners. Marjorie had learned so well from her mom that she started working some "magic" in her dealings with her daddy. She never lied but said things that got a nod from her father. That was big nowadays. Daddy looked terrible. Marjorie guessed he looked at least sixty years old, maybe even seventy. He was very thin now and ate like a guppy. When Marjorie asked how he was feeling, he usually said that he had a bad headache. She always said she was sorry that he didn't feel well. Sometimes she would offer to rub his neck. Occasionally, he would say okay. Marjorie knew this helped keep things calm. This was for the betterment of her mother, not her father.

One day Marjorie received a letter from Sarah. In the letter, she explained that her husband wanted Sarah to focus on them as a married couple, not her family. He was her husband; he actually demanded to be the focus. Sarah had no choice. It would be okay to write letters from time to time, but visits would be restricted to once a year. Marjorie knew this was a result of Daddy not giving the young couple money and cutting them off. Sarah's husband had been furious that they had not received any help when they really needed it. How could a family with immense wealth not help? He was still mad. Marjorie and Abigail knew restricting Sarah's visits was payback – how very sad for the three women. Sarah did also mention that they were expecting.

By the time, Marjorie was eighteen, her family was in disarray. There had been no contact from Henry for almost two years. A pregnant sister, who needed her family's support and help, couldn't visit but once a year at her husband's approval. A father, who was acting like a dictator, and a mother, somewhat broken by the whole mess, couldn't be in the same room without the tension going through the roof. They never talked. The only person doing well was Marjorie.

Marjorie was getting along with Daddy to a degree. Abigail was starting to laugh in conversations with her friends and Marjorie. TWO STABS IN THE HEART COULD NOT KEEP HER DOWN. Abigail was strong and resilient. Daughter and mom were having their talks again. Marjorie had nurtured her mother back from the abyss by using the same lessons her mother had taught her. Her key focus every day was to do good deeds and be positive. Marjorie had become someone very special.

Marjorie's friends knew of her situation. M was Marjorie's nickname at school with all her friends. She loved it as she saw it as a sign of affection, and this was exactly the case. Marjorie had found her calling during the creation of the first talent show. Everyone knew M couldn't sing or dance. She was the most popular person at the tryouts, and some, in such a position, would have tried to push their way into the show but not Marjorie. One day everyone was talking about the opening act.

M quickly spoke, "Well, if I were the opening act, I would empty the theater." She laughed and went on, "Maybe I could do the closing act. It would make the rest of you look so amazing. You all are so great. You are all kind not to make fun of my stage skills. I love you all for that, but I want you all to know that I am aware of my lack of skill." She smiled again. "It makes me so aware of how wonderful you all are. I will do whatever I can to help."

Marjorie was fantastic at getting things done. She organized, motivated, encouraged, and made the production lively and fun. One day at practice, things weren't going particularly well. Marjorie gathered the performers together.

M said, "Everybody knows each of you has so much talent. Each of you is different, and that is a wonderful thing. This is exactly what the audience wants to see. Individual performers doing things in their own style. Embrace your style. The audience will love it, every bit of it, even a mistake or two. The audience wants to see you having fun. Okay?" From that moment on, every day at practice, M led chants, "FUN, FUN, FUN, LET'S HAVE SOME FUN – FUN, FUN, FUN, and LET'S HAVE SOME FUN." Marjorie always danced as she sang. Everyone enjoyed the moment led by their very special leader.

Every couple of days, M might say something like, "Well, if someone gets sick, I'll fill in. I know all the words, as I am such a fan of all you talented performers. Wouldn't it be fun if I could do several numbers?" Then she would smile and say, "I love you guys."

All the people at practice loved Marjorie. Who wouldn't? A bright, beautiful girl who could laugh at herself. Everyone knew she was the most important part of the show, but M didn't. She only wanted to help make the talent show a success. Performing good deeds and being positive gave me so much joy. Her mother had made it abundantly clear over the years that helping others is the greatest thing a person can do.

When Marjorie started college, she entered as a strong and positive young woman. She carried her mother's lessons with her. M studied very hard as her daddy was paying for it. She figured that her daddy hadn't mentioned the elite school that Sarah went to, probably, because Marjorie was the only person who was friendly to him at home. He needed someone. It would please him that his daughter was not only beautiful but also bright. It might also help the situation at home. Marjorie knew there were no longer any family dinners. Her mother and she wrote letters back and forth often. Once again, they were delivered through one of Abigail's friends. Marjorie knew her parents would not divorce, as it would damage the family name and daddy's business.

During Marjorie's senior year, her daddy died. His doctor told Abigail later that he had advised her husband to take some time off to get his health back in order, but he refused. On the final day of his life, Daddy got angry at work and was yelling at some people in his office. Rumor had it that they had lost the company quite a bit of money. Daddy screamed for them to get out of the building. He told them they were all fired; they wouldn't find any jobs in this city. They found him on the floor several hours later.

Thomas had been involved with M for three months. They were already scheduled to be married in three months. Marjorie left school to go home for a while to handle all the arrangements. Abigail had no access to any of the estate, so M quickly arranged to get enough money to handle the final dealings with her daddy. Marjorie had met with daddy's lawyer. She arranged for the will to be read along with any legal ramifications. In a short time, the lawyer became a fan. He was so impressed with M's mannerisms, looks, and that wonderful smile. He was very helpful. The lawyer explained many things and even some items that he probably should not have. He did mention that her father was a difficult client. Marjorie smiled as she reached over and touched his arm and said, "You should have lived with him." The reply came back, "No thank you."

She fired the household staff explaining delicately that they had worked for her father, and he was gone. Regretfully, their services were no longer needed. She did give them a small severance pay. It was only right. They were only following orders. Abigail quickly hired a very small staff to assist her around the estate. Marjorie handled all the money. At no time were Sarah or her mother involved with finances. Abigail was adamant about this, as she did not trust daddy's lawyer. Marjorie knew everything was going to be okay because he had told her what to do and how to do it.

Thomas was there for much of the time. He assisted where he could, talked to lawyers, supported M in all her dealings, and provided a pleasant demeanor. His wonderful sense of humor was on display around the house when he was there. It was much appreciated. Abigail absolutely loved Thomas. She told Marjorie that she could not be happier for them; they were very special together. She also told me that she had met someone.

There were two quick lessons for Marjorie from her mother during her stay at home while making all the arrangements. Abigail started out by saying that she apologized for her comments about wealth. They might have been too harsh. She explained that wealth sometimes corrupts one's soul. Wealth becomes who they are; it is all that really matters.

Your father was that way. He damaged many people on his way to wealth, and it didn't bother him in the slightest.

Abigail spoke slowly as she took Marjorie's hand, "Because of what he did, it caused me to shun wealth to a large degree. After our talk, I realized that I had made too strong of an argument against showing off your wealth to others; I apologize. I still don't like the flaunting part or the arrogance, but people who make money honestly and help people along the way should be able to enjoy it. The lesson I am getting at is we simply should always reflect on our words. We know when our words are spoken in a strong or harsh manner. In doing so, a person's sense of right and wrong will alert them that they might have gotten something wrong. If so, they need to correct it as quickly as possible. Again, I apologize. A quick story about a wonderful man, and I will let you talk, my dear sweet daughter."

"Many years ago your father had a business deal with a rancher north of here. I had met the man in a previous meeting, and we really had a pleasant conversation. Your father wanted me to go along to help with the deal. I went along but had no plans to intervene on your father's behalf. When we arrived at this fine restaurant, the rancher was already sitting at the table. When he stood to greet us, he had on the same type of clothes as last time, a flannel shirt, overalls, and cowboy boots. I stated that it was so pleasant to see him again.

"He smiled at me, took my hand, and addressed my husband, 'I'm sorry that we won't be having dinner tonight. There's no need, as I am not selling you that land that we previously discussed. I am a good businessperson; I do my homework. It is just not going to work out. Again, I am sorry, but I wanted to tell you to your face. If you need to know more, we can ask your lovely wife to explore the fantastic gardens outside as we have a drink at the bar. I can quickly explain my reasons." "I knew what was coming next.

"Your father said to the rancher that a drink sounded like a good idea. The rancher apologized to me for the inconvenience, but the nice man explained that he personally didn't mind because he has to see the most beautiful woman he had ever met again. He smiled and nodded his head. I meandered outside to some of the most beautiful landscapes that I had ever seen. Your father was there in five minutes and simply said, 'Let's go".

"I'm telling you this story because the gentleman we met that evening was one of the richest men in the Midwest. He told me at our last dinner together that he was a small rancher when he started out as a young man. He had a code of behavior that he lived by, and no amount of money would ever change who he was. I believe the rancher probably told your father that your daddy was a smart person, aggressive, knowledgeable, but he wasn't honest. Therefore, the rancher couldn't do business with him. He probably finished with the words, 'I'm sorry once again, but this needed to be said in person. Good night to you.' Then he would have walked away. Now it's your time to talk, my precious."

"Well, my dearest mother, my moral compass is well established because of you; I love you for that. It led me right to the man that I love very much. Thomas and I talk so much about helping people. Mom, he is the kindest man I have ever met. We agree on many philosophical ideals; we will do good things together. I have always been amazed at how wonderful of a person you have been throughout your marriage. You never let Daddy change who you are. By the way, I am very impressed with the rancher you met with Daddy. That is exactly the kind of people I would want Thomas and I to be if we were rich. I can see how both the rancher and Daddy may have influenced you concerning your comments about wealth. Mother, I still feel the same way I did earlier when we discussed flaunting your wealth. That will never be Thomas and I. Thomas says that I am a very special woman. I won't bore you with how he went on and on, but he really had quite a few things to say."

"Mother," Marjorie started crying but went on, "thank you for the hundreds of hours of talks. You shaped me into the person I am, and I love who I am. Words cannot describe the amount of love and respect I have for you. I can only hope to do half as well as you in shaping my children." She took her mother's hands, squeezed them gently, and kissed her on the cheek.

Abigail inched closer to her daughter, gave her a long hug, and whispered to her, "You will be wonderful in many ways. You and Thomas will do good deeds, spread kindness and warmth to those you meet in contact with, but, above all, you will share a love and tenderness with your family that will enrich their lives tremendously. I am so very happy for you."

Chapter 5

the Teaching Team

Nate's learning from the Smiths began well before he quit school to join them at the Smith's Veterinary Clinic and Gardening Seminar. Nate was a champion observer. In his interactions with the Smiths at town gatherings, he was so impressed at how much they smiled and laughed. These two facial expressions usually were connected to words. Nate knew if he wanted to smile and laugh like the Smiths, he would have to talk more. Talking would have to come first. After getting comfortable with that, he could learn to smile and laugh. He really enjoyed watching the Smiths laugh, smile, and have fun.

This was something that he thought he should try. His mother was also very good at smiling and laughing, and she was a great talker. Unfortunately, she was very busy with Nate's younger brother and sister. Nate didn't want to take up her time although he knew she would volunteer 100%. The Smiths had the time, especially Mrs. Smith. The Smiths were also very kind. Maybe they might help Nate become more social, express himself in a more friendly fashion, and enjoy people in general. Nate knew from his parents and by his scores at school that he was smart. Why couldn't he enjoy people like his parents and the Smiths?

Nate knew that he had to change, and one day Mrs. Smith explained to Nate, "Learning takes place over time. Sometimes it takes many baby steps to learn a skill." Nate had heard the exact words from his mother. Mrs. Smith continued, "When I was newly married to Thomas, we decided to cook a meal for his parents whom we were living with at the time. We cooked for about an hour and followed all the instructions. We were so proud of ourselves. We sat down for dinner, and everything was terrible. I still remember very vividly, what Thomas' dad, Bart, said when he was asked how he liked the meal. He said, 'The water was very good.' We all laughed until we cried. To this very day, if something goes bad, Thomas will ask me if I need a glass of water, and, yes, we still laugh about it. By the way,

Thomas' mother, Millie, taught me how to cook, and I have been told I am good. It just took a little time. Millie was a wonderful teacher and is a very special woman. I appreciate her so much. Nate, be patient with your learning. Please remember that laughing with someone, never at someone, makes almost everything better and learning takes place over time."

When Nate left the town gathering that day with his parents, he was thinking about Mrs. Smith. He sure enjoyed getting the lessons from her today. He didn't exactly know what it was about her, but he felt she was the one person who could help him learn to be more comfortable around people. He had never enjoyed a person's company as much as he did Mrs. Smith's – not even his mother's. He remembered her words, "Nate, I really enjoyed visiting with you today. If I can help you with any questions you might have, feel free to ask anytime. Okay?" When she said okay to Nate, she reached out and held his hands for a moment. Nate felt something, a rapid heartbeat, shortness of breath, and/or a buzz in the brain. He didn't know what it was exactly, but he felt something, a strong sensation. He also felt a strong connection to Mrs. Smith. She had felt the same feeling.

Nate enjoyed school, but he especially liked it when Mrs. Smith took over for the day. He remembered many things she did to teach a lesson. One day she explained that the class was going to have a math test tomorrow. She explained that she would grade the tests during lunch and hand out prizes for the top boy and girl scorer's right after lunch.

"Teachers always want their students to study hard and do their best on any test," Mrs. Smith said. She continued speaking slowly, "Well, class," she paused, "will you please study hard and do your best? I want each of you to promise me right now that you will. Please nod your heads if you'll do it for me, your parents, and yourselves." Everyone nodded, even the kids who weren't good at math. That is how much everyone liked Mrs. Smith. She continued, "We will clap for the winners and all say GOOD JOB – WELL DONE."

The next day some students were excited about the big test; some were nervous. Miss Bridgeman never spoke to the class about studying hard as if Mrs. Smith did. Nate really enjoyed her speech. He never saw the class so motivated. There was an equal number of boys and girls in class. After the test was graded, Mrs. Smith gave the top boy and girl eight cookies each. The class and Mrs. Smith clapped for the winners and said "GOOD JOB – WELL DONE." The winners seemed to be very proud because the praise was genuine. Nate was impressed that everybody worked so hard on the test.

Then the lesson began. As the top scorers handed out a rather large cookie to each student, Mrs. Smith explained, "Everyone wins in regards to this test. You all worked hard. Everybody studied and concentrated to the best of their ability. I couldn't be prouder of all of you. You are all winners. Don't you all agree that everybody in the class wins? Thank you all for doing so well." As the class enjoyed the tasty cookies, Mrs. Smith handed back the tests, thanking each student for their big effort.

Some students may have missed the true lesson, but not Nate. Encourage and reward good effort. This makes the person feel good about the work they have done and want to do better next time. Nate had never seen the class so happy after a test. This was a lesson that Nate never forgot.

There was one more lesson Mrs. Smith taught that Nate thought was so great. He even shared it with his parents. It started out by Mrs. Smith saying that she wasn't sure it was her job to be teaching this lesson, but she was going to do it. She would ask for forgiveness if she had to. A map of the United States was in the front of the room on top of the chalkboard. It had been pulled down as Mrs. Smith started to talk. When she raised it up, the students could see the following:

1. You have four eyes.
2. My hair is prettier than yours is.
3. You are no good.
4. I am the smartest kid in class.

5. You people are losers.
6. I am going to beat you up.
7. You look weird.

"You students have said these things to each other today. It hurts my heart to hear such things," she said with watery eyes. She continued, "Your words should never be disrespectful. There should never be victims from your words." She paused for a while and then said, "You didn't know did you? Your bragging words and belittling words can make victims of your classmates. I am sure you did not mean to hurt your classmates' feelings. I am going to put two rules on the side of the room. I want you to say the rules to yourself every day when you come into class. Okay?"

Later that day the words, SHOW RESPECT AND BE KIND, were on the side of the room. The next day they were gone when the students arrived. Miss Bridgeman had taken them down. She didn't like the way Mrs. Smith taught school. She wasn't trained and did things inappropriately according to Miss Bridgeman. For example, Mrs. Smith let the students work together by grade level in math. Helping each other is a good thing according to Mrs. Smith, but make sure you are helping the learning, not distracting from it. The students seemed to enjoy it, but Miss Bridgeman said there was too much talking and not enough work. She also thought giving out prizes was just plain wrong. The students quietly disagreed.

When the Johnsons heard about the lesson about words given by Mrs. Smith, as told by their son, they were both impressed. They liked the idea that words shouldn't be hurtful. Mrs. Johnson mentioned that in listening to the Smiths over the last eight years, she could not remember any harmful words ever coming from their lips. These two people really did practice what Mrs. Smith had said in her lesson: SHOW RESPECT – BE KIND.

Mr. Johnson spoke, "I'm going to ask Marjorie if I could use part of her lesson in one of my sermons. I am sure she will say 'yes' as long as I don't use her name. You know she never wants credit for anything."

A short time later after Nate had traveled with Dr. Smith on a large number of "business" calls; he noticed the doctor constantly treated his customers with respect and kindness. He would say things like: "Let's take another look at this, okay?", "We can fix this, don't you think?", or "If we work together we'll make her as good as new, okay?"

Dr. Smith used the word "we" an awful lot. Nate thought it made people comfortable and part of a team. Thomas never said things like, "You screwed up", "You forgot", or things that put the blame on the customer. Dr. Smith explained to Nate, "The customer feels bad already, and you should never make them feel worse. We are there to help. In fact, remember that when dealing with people in general. You don't need to hurt people's feelings when trying to help them."

Years later when Nate was in a conversation with Marjorie, she explained, "My Thomas is the kindest person I've ever known. He is also the smartest." Nate liked the words, my Thomas; he thought that was special.

Nate also noticed that Dr. Smith really treated all the animals he doctored very carefully. He knew they were of great value to the owners. He was always concerned if the animal went down for a while or couldn't work anymore. Many times, he would be involved in helping to replace an animal that could no longer work. Thomas explained to Nate that these animals provide the labor to grow the product. Without the animals, there is no revenue source. Nate, it wouldn't be right if we didn't help our neighbor.

Dr. Smith was constantly sharing his knowledge, humor, and life lessons with Nate. They traveled many miles in a buggy to and from many customers, and Nate couldn't ever remember lulls in the conversation. By eighteen, Nate was stronger than Dr. Smith was and did most of the heavy work, including delivering any of the large stock they handled. Dr. Smith knew Nate could do most of any work they came across. He had been a vet in training for seven years and knew so much. Thomas was so proud.

Marjorie and Thomas decided that it was time to teach Nate about the power of giving. Thomas would do the teaching as Nate had observed the kind vet giving to so many over the years. Thomas told Nate one day, "My dad said that giving was one of the greatest things a person can do, but he seldom ever used the word giving. Dad explained that many people do not want to be given anything; it is against their nature. He always used the word help in place of give. It seemed to work better. Words like 'we could really help each other' or 'It would really help me if' made it much easier for my dad to give a neighbor a helping hand." One of Thomas' favorite ones that was used by his dad many times was, "You'd be doing me a huge favor by taking this horse off my hands. I have three horses already, and this one just gets in the way, not to mention the cost and upkeep. Please take him. You'd really be helping me out."

Thomas finished the lesson off by telling Nate that many times the person receiving the help ends up giving to others. Many times these recipients of the "helping hand" also become givers. It is easy to see the multiplying effect of giving. Don't ever forget the power of giving.

Nate thanked Thomas for this great lesson. "I've never really thought about the power of giving; it's really amazing. If you teach a teenager to give as if you are doing to me, they could give to so many over their lifetime. When these folks, in turn, give to others, the multiplying effect would be amazing. I would need a journal to keep track of the giving." He smiled.

Thomas returned the smile and said, "It's great that you keep a journal, but, my greatest apprentice, you won't need to keep count. You will feel wonderful inside; doing God's will generates such inner happiness. It is truly a blessing."

Mrs. Smith and Nate worked around the property. She taught him so much about gardening. He learned more about supplements, pruning, and how and when to water. Nate thought he knew quite a bit about gardening prior to working with the Smiths, but Marjorie taught him more. She also supervised his weekly lessons in school. She taught history, some math, literature, and English composition. He enjoyed both aspects of his days with Mrs. Smith. She even taught him how to cook. She said that every man needs to be able to do some things in a kitchen. She stated that Thomas was quite good. Above all, Marjorie taught by example. Nate watched, listened, and learned just by being with this amazing woman.

One day when Nate was twelve, he cut a rather large root when he was cultivating. He felt terrible, but Marjorie explained that mistakes are part of life. Everybody makes them, but you will make less, as you grow older. Age, experience, and learning will help you cut down on mistakes. She showed him how to trim the broken root to promote new growth. She continued to explain to Nate that being remorseful and apologizing are two key fixes in repairing mistakes. They need to be done immediately. These two things will make everybody feel better about the mistake. It will also help you to learn from it. No one likes it when someone makes the same mistake repeatedly unless there is a good reason for it. Nate quickly apologized; Mrs. Smith could tell by his facial expression that Nate was very remorseful.

The number of Nate's mistakes did definitely go down rather quickly in the next few years, but he always remembered to apologize. Nate hated to make mistakes, so he was remorseful every time. He always added the question, "What can I do to make this better?" He had learned that from Mrs. Smith on the few mistakes she made during the lessons. Nate suspected that she made the mistakes on purpose to reinforce her lesson on mistakes. Nate loved Marjorie's lessons.

One afternoon when Nate was fourteen and a half, Marjorie explained how wonderfully Nate was progressing in all aspects of his learning. "Thomas says you are a tremendous help and can diagnose many situations. GOOD FOR YOU. You have done so well in your school lessons. I always give the student with the highest grades an A+. You are that student. Congratulations, I'm giving you the highest grade in the class, an A+."

Nate smiled and quickly countered, "And I always give the best teacher in the class an A+!" They both laughed.

Marjorie then explained to Nate that there was one assignment that she wanted to give to him, and she wanted him to get another A+ on it. Nate replied that he would do his best. She went on to explain, "I want you to know how amazing your father and mother are. I love your parents for being who they are. Your father loves you, and it shows in all the words he has for you and in all the work, you two share. Cherish your time with him. I know he does.

He loves you very much."

"In my opinion, a mother's love may be even deeper than a father's. It may be God's way. For when a child is very young, the baby and mother are bonded for life. I know you don't hug much. I have seen you hug your mom back when she hugs you. I wish for you, I pray for you, to show your parents the love you have for them in some form: a note, a few words, a gift, or maybe a hug. I want you to hug your mother more often. I want you to initiate the hug. This will make her so happy. It would also be a great example for your younger brother and sister to see. Can you do that?"

Nate didn't say a word. He walked over to Marjorie and gave her a hug, a long one. Then he kissed her cheek and said, "I'll try." Marjorie's eyes watered. She couldn't talk.

One day when the outside work was done, Marjorie and Nate were having a long lunch that included a lesson on communication. Marjorie explained that words are a powerful tool. She reminded Nate of Thomas Paine. He knew all about him as he had done a written report on him for history.

"Good," she said; she paused; then continued, "So you know all about written communication and how it's mightier than the sword. Many people do not realize this. Business letters, written communication to friends, and romantic intimacies expressed through the pen are samples of powerful written communication. I have a box in the bedroom full of letters from my mother, friends, and Thomas. They mean the world to me; I read them often. I also have some legal documents in another box. They are critically important. Some have been used in court and will be used again in the future. Please remember the importance of written communication. Nate, you are a wonderful writer, so I don't want you to forget your skill. Use it with your family, friends, or maybe someone special in your life."

The mentor continued, "Oral communication, another form of relating to others, can be extremely difficult to master. There are no rewrites. Words spoken are out in the air to be heard by all. Some seem to have a gift at it. Thomas is a champion at it. Listen to him and learn. We must always be careful with our words. This is a very difficult task. The wrong words can be hurtful and even devastating to some, especially children. Bragging is something I am not fond of. It can be somewhat arrogant, possibly unkind, or sometimes disrespectful. Enough said. I know you'll never be a person who does such a thing."

"Over the past several years, I have asked you many questions. It was not to because you stress, but instead, it was for you to practice your talking skills. As if I have said many times, practice makes perfect. You are so much better now because we have shared so many hours of conversation, and I want you to know that I have enjoyed our talks very much. Thank you, Nate. Thomas tells me that he is always aware of the people he is talking to. Never does he forget that. In doing so, he doesn't embarrass or belittle any of his customers. We have never had that problem between us, but you always need to be careful. That's the purpose of this lesson today." Marjorie asked Nate a question, "Nate, is it easier talking to me now as compared to four years ago?"

"Oh, very much so," replied a smiling Nate. "I actually enjoy the talks. Thank you, my teacher and mentor."

Marjorie smiled and nodded; she knew she had done well so far. It felt so good. She went on to explain to Nate that when people talk to each other over time, they create a bond. A friendship may ensue, or, in the case of a young couple, romance may be a possibility. She told Nate that this was part of being human. She thanked him for helping to build the bond that they now share.

As Nate walked home, he was thinking that he really enjoyed the bond he shared with his primary mentor; having a bond with someone is special. Nate never forgot this thought...

Chapter 6

More Lessons

One day when Nate was sixteen, Marjorie decided it was time to finish the communication lesson. Nate was going to work with Thomas at a few ranches in the afternoon. Mrs. Smith gave Nate a homework assignment. She had previously explained what some of the effects of oral communication were and now Nate was to look for any of them on his trip to the ranches. Marjorie and Nate would finish the lesson tomorrow after Nate reported his findings.

The next morning while working in the garden, Nate explained what he observed. Words seem to affect a person has face the most. The eyebrows and forehead seemed to work as one; the eyes and the mouth seemed to be the keys. He explained what negative words did to facial expressions and the opposite, kind or positive words. Nate said that he had been aware of words and their effect on facial expressions. He mentioned that his father sometimes used negative words to teach a lesson. He saw the facial expressions of Doris and Andy. It always bothered Nate to see them on his brother and sister after their father's negative words but knew that is how you learn.

He continued that it had never occurred to him until this morning that his mother often used a different method to address any wrongdoings. It took more time, more patience, and some dialogue. It worked very well and usually ended with a pat on the back or a hug. Nate could understand both methods. Nate informed Marjorie that his brother and sister most often had joyous and happy expressions on their faces from his parents' lessons. "My parents support, praise, encourage, and smile during lessons, and when this happens, the looks on my brother's and sister's faces make me so happy. I love it during these types of lessons," said a smiling Nate.

Marjorie listened carefully to Nate's words because she enjoyed his progress at expressing himself so much, but she had to excuse herself to finish some cooking she had started just before Nate arrived.

When she returned, Nate said that he had seen his father and mother use different techniques to teach a lesson when my brother or sister do something wrong. He wondered which one was better. He asked his mentor.

Marjorie finished off the lesson by saying, "Nate, both methods are good. I am not telling you one is better than the other is. You can use both. I am sure your parents use both. What I want you to always do is to be constantly aware of your words. Do no harm, unless you think it is necessary. Oral communication is a beautiful tool that allows us to achieve so much. Business success, friendship, teaching, and love are a few, but I repeat, oral communication can do great damage. Always beware of your words."

Marjorie planned to discuss unspoken and/or special communication, but felt she had spent enough time on communication at this time. Nate had enough to digest. She would spend time reinforcing written and oral communication and leave this other two for later. She had a plan for Nate and her. It would be very different, very fun, and involve two simple lessons that she truly hoped Nate would enjoy. She asked, "Nate, can you come over tomorrow at 7:30 in the morning? I would like us to go to Potterville on the stage. It leaves between 7:45 and 8 a.m. Wear nice clothes. Thomas will join us for an early dinner and drive us home."

Nate smiled and said, "Yes, that sounds like lots of fun."

The next day they did go to Potterville and spent some time visiting different establishments. Marjorie showed Nate her favorite places; they ate lunch at one. After lunch, Mrs. Smith rented a buggy to go to a small lake just outside of town. In addition, a gorgeous little creek fed the lake. They both thoroughly enjoyed the scenery as they visited with one another. Thomas met them later at a nice restaurant in town where they enjoyed a splendid dinner. They were on their way home shortly after 5:00. The ride, as usual, was very enjoyable.

Nate surprised Marjorie by his words when they reached home. He said, as he shook Thomas' hand, "Thank you for dinner. It was great food and great conversation. Thank you for traveling so far and bringing us home." Nate then walked over to Marjorie, gave her a big hug, and spoke with some emotion, "This was an awesome day. Thank you for the wonderful conversation; it was more than great."

"You're very welcome, Nate. It was my pleasure," whispered Mrs. Smith, as she did not want her voice to crack. She was a little emotional from such a fantastic day with her "son".

The next day Marjorie explained to Nate that even though yesterday was so much fun, there were two small lessons involved, small talk and relaxation. The two are often intertwined. These two things are often done when we are with friends, family, and always done when we are on a date. They are a critical part of any courtship and an active part of any long-term relationship. She then asked Nate if he had enjoyed the small talk.

"I didn't think it was small talk at all," said Nate. "I enjoyed every part of it, especially learning more things about you."

"That's because we are family," replied Marjorie. Nate did not respond; he just nodded his head and smiled.

When Nate was seventeen, Marjorie totally surprised him one day while sharing a lunch prepared by Nate's mother. She started out by saying, "Nate, I have some interesting news. You have learned everything I have to teach. You scored another A+ in my book. I have, of course, explained all this to Thomas. We are as very proud of you as I am sure your parents are. I'm going to ask you to do something from time to time if you are willing?"

Nate quickly replied, "Sure, it isn't ironing Thomas' shirts, is it?"

Marjorie laughed and replied, "No, but it involves you sharing with me some knowledge that you're going to learn from some of Thomas' books. He says you are ready for a couple of college text books on veterinary medicine."

Nate laughed and said, "You want me to be the teacher and you the student?"

Marjorie answered, "Yes, won't that be fun? I hope you're an easy grader?"

The young man answered, "Mr. Johnson still gives the top scholar an A+. He also gives the same grade to the two people who exhibit the most kindness or respect towards others. Wouldn't it be great if you won all three? It's never been done before."

Marjorie didn't answer. She gave Nate a hug while she was thinking how much Nate's words sounded just like something her dear Thomas would have said. She would have to tell him later. He would love it.

Over the next two years, Nate and Marjorie shared the job of teacher. Of course, Marjorie still did most of the teaching. She talked about social skills and some philosophy, along with a review of things she had previously taught. She was constantly asking Nate questions and was intrigued, not only by the length of Nate's responses but also by the content. She was able to see the influence of Thomas and Mary in his words, and, yes, she was able to see herself in most of Nate's responses. This gave her immense pleasure.

Nate's lessons were a little rough at first. Marjorie explained that delivering a lesson is very difficult. She assured Nate that he would be wonderful in his presentations if he continued to practice. The more lessons you give, the better you will get. She said that she really enjoyed his delivery, the smiles, and, most of all, any jokes he included. The smiles and jokes mean you are comfortable with your student. She smiled. It was Thomas' idea for Nate to present these lessons to Marjorie. He had thought that Nate was ready for this advanced development.

The Smiths were concerned that it would be too much for Nate, but both adults were closely monitoring his progress. He had come so far in answering questions or reporting information that he discovered during his years of lessons from the Smiths. Initiating and creating the dialogue to present a lesson was a big jump for their diligent student. The Smiths both agreed that, at this time, Nate was progressing well and seemed to be enjoying it. What they didn't know was Nate would do anything for the Smiths. He was always motivated to do well.

One morning Marjorie explained to Nate, "Tomorrow you'll be busy all day with Thomas doing a few ranch and farm visits in the morning and the annual animal auction in the afternoon. I won't see you all day except to say 'Good morning' when I see you first thing in the morning, but I do have an assignment for you. You can do two things at the same time."

"Oh, great, I get to multi-task," said Nate. "My mother is very good at it; my father says he's terrible at it."

"Women, many times, do handle different tasks at the same time. When a woman has children, she has to. I believe God has given women this skill because they need it," explained Marjorie. "Men can do it also if they really try. Thomas can do it, and I'm sure you'll learn the skill also."

Nate jumped in with, "Don't tell me; all it takes is practice and more practice."

Marjorie laughed and said, "Thank you for listening to my lessons. How many times have I said those very words?" She smiled.

A smiling Nate replied, "Enough times that I made a plague saying SUCCESS TAKES PRACTICE AND MORE PRACTICE."

"Oh, can I see it?" asked Marjorie.

"Sure," said Nate, "next time you come to dinner I'll have Andy show it to you. I gave it to him last year, so he could benefit from it. I sure did."

"That's wonderful!" exclaimed Marjorie. "Sharing your key to success with your brother is very thoughtful of you. Now, your assignment for the day is simple. You are to watch people and observe how much they smile. You don't need to write anything down but keep an eye out for people's smiles and the ensuing interactions. We'll talk about your findings tomorrow."

Nate smiled and touched Marjorie's shoulder as he started to leave, telling Marjorie, "I've never had a smiling assignment before."

Thomas interjected as he was hugging his wife, "When I see Marjorie every morning, she makes me smile. I must be her smiling assignment." All three were smiling as the men left.

As Mrs. Smith sipped on a cup of coffee, she thought about what had just transpired.

Nate surely did converse with a great skill that included smiles and laughs initiated by him. He was truly someone special. All of a sudden, she had the utmost need to write Mary a note. In the note, she wrote that it was not normally her place to praise herself or take credit for anything she helped with, but her seeing and hearing Nate this morning filled her with so much emotion. She needed to share this. Marjorie asked Mary if she would like to come for tea and pastry. It would be so much fun to share some more Nate stories.

Three days later the two women shared stories. It was heartfelt with handkerchiefs out. Mary ended the visit with these words, "I have a rather long narrative for you. I like to think of a child as a frame of a house. As they grow and learn from their many teachers, they end up being a completed house. With good teaching, hard work, and the right intellect, the house will be wonderful. As you know, not all houses are as such. Sometimes the right child can build the house by itself, but it is rather difficult. With average input, the house may, very likely, be average. I want to be adamant when I say that there is nothing wrong with average. Most average people achieve status and success through hard work, a solid family, and a good lifestyle. Most everybody is average. It is not a bad thing. My dear Marjorie, we have built a three story spectacular mansion.

"You and Thomas have engineered and constructed most of it during the last seven and a half years. I was a formal builder myself for four years before my marriage, so I, more than most, appreciate the unbelievable mentoring by you and Thomas. You, my idol in so many ways, are the most amazing person I have ever known. Our son always had the intellect and work ethic, but he needed special care and teaching to reach complete success in his growth. You were the guiding light and captain of the building crew that led him to where he is today. He will do many great things in his life. He may be your greatest achievement. He loves you so much."

With a few tears rolling down her face, Marjorie walked over to Mary as the visitor stood to say goodbye. Marjorie took Mary's hands in hers and gently squeezed them. As they said goodbye with a long embrace, Mary said, "I love you, M."

"I love you, M2," was the response.

After M2 left, Marjorie sat there thinking about Nate. She was very happy with the man she helped create. She knew it was her greatest work; Thomas felt the same way. Nate's comments a couple of days ago about smiles showed so much about his growth. He had explained that smiles seem quite powerful. They have an immediate positive effect on others. Many times a smile creates more smiles. He mentioned that smiles should be in a medical journal because they seem to be contagious. M liked it when he said that smiling when you first see someone often makes that person feel like you value them. Smiling as you visit with a friend shows that you are enjoying their company. PROFOUND He thanked Marjorie for the lesson as he smiled. He promised to smile as often as he could. He then gave her a hug along with a kiss on the cheek. WOW!

When Nate was nineteen, Marjorie explained one day that over the last eight years she and Nate shared what she called unspoken communication. Special looks, certain touches, and different types of movement convey an unspoken communication. She explained, "Hugging someone communicates to that person; Smiling and laughing do the same. I could name more, but I think you understand. Nate, I have enjoyed the many unspoken communications between us over the years. Thank you so very much. They were and are very special to me. I am sure your family feels the same way. I am not talking about negative unspoken communication. You know what that is, and I choose not to discuss that. I truly hope that you will always focus on positive communication, whether it's verbal or nonverbal."

"Thomas and I have a wonderful type of unspoken communication. It makes our marriage so much better than if we didn't have it. I hope for you that one day you will find someone with whom you can share this wonderful type of communication. One more thing," she paused and then said, "Thomas and I have special words that we share only between ourselves. I can't even tell you because they wouldn't be special any longer. This special communication or words if you like, help create that ultimate bond that couples share. This sense of togetherness can lead to a deep and lasting love. I hope for you, my dear boy, that one day you will find that special person to share such a type of communication. Can I have a hug?"

As Nate and Marjorie embraced, Nate spoke, "So there are four types of communication; all seem to be powerful in one way or another. Thank you for these lessons. I will do my best to be positive." Marjorie did not say a word. She simply hugged Nate a little harder and kissed him on the cheek.

Chapter 7

A Completed House

When Nate was twenty years old, he worked in the garden with Mrs. Smith sitting in a chair discussing a multitude of topics with her favorite student. She was always smiling and laughing, praising Nate's work, or asking him questions on various topics. There were also many days when Nate went on calls to customers without Thomas. Nate knew that something was not right, and he knew it was Marjorie. While she talked and visited in the morning like always, after lunch, she took a nap while Nate continued with the chores.

Thomas was much quieter than normal. Then one day Thomas was back to his normal self. Nate found out later that Marjorie had taught Thomas a lesson. A lesson that Nate would receive in writing sometime later.

Marjorie had explained to Thomas, "My mother taught me this lesson as her time was growing shorter. She explained that you never judge a life well lived by its length, years on the job, or the money earned. If a man lives in prison until the age of eighty, did he have a good life? If a man makes huge amounts of money but has no friends or family, has he had a good life? Money is nice, but it is not the key to a good life. Work is good, but it isn't the answer either. In her opinion, these things don't matter in the end. If a woman has not had a chance to enhance her skills and embrace that emotional bond to others that women seem to inherit from their maker, has she lived a good life? Sadly, she has not. There are many people in this world who die without knowing the pleasures of a life well lived."

My mother also stated, "If money, work, or longevity of life aren't the keys to a life well lived, then what is? The answer involves other people. When a person's time to meet their maker nears, this individual should reflect on the memories they have stored in their mind. I hope that the memories are full of family and friends. If these memories are positive and show support for others, there will be a feeling of contentment. If the person shared laughs, smiles, and love with others, these relationships give them a feeling of warmth."

"If a person accomplishes a lifetime of doing good things within their means, they feel contentment and warmth. If they leave behind a legacy of kindness and respect, they realize they made a positive difference in people's lives. This warms people's souls and helps prepare them for their last journey."

"Rich people who have abused others along the way, accomplished wealth through devious and ruthless means, or placed money over friendship, don't have these wonderful feelings that come from helping others. Lawbreakers who have hurt people during their lifetime often feel remorse for their dastardly deeds. There is no contentment and warmth in these people's hearts. There's often sadness as they reflect on their past."

"If a person supported their friends and family in any way they could, it should comfort them that they did well with the people close to them. Above all, the love of a family, both receiving and giving, is the keystone of a life well lived. Everyone should do all the items mentioned previously with family. In doing so, the love that radiates outward from each person in the family touches everyone nearby."

"This love and many other aspects of support prepare young folks to possibly reach a great contributing factor of a life well lived, the love of a spouse. Our creator has provided the opportunity for two people to possibly reach this highest emotional bond. It is not likely without the ingredients of respect and appreciation, smiles and laughs, positive interaction and support, kindness and love, and the special interactions that cement a bond that becomes the pinnacle of human interaction. All of these things are enhanced by the value each person feels for the other. This bonded relationship is the foundation that leads to many accomplishments that determine a life well lived."

"It should be mentioned that individuals can also accomplish many things that would qualify them to have lived a life well lived. It very likely would be somewhat more difficult for them to succeed in these supportive and positive endeavors, and this is why these individuals should be especially proud of their work. Their friends and family would be so fortunate to have witnessed such good things."

"So in our last days on this earth, value what has made your life worthy of a life well lived. Nobody has had a perfect life, but if you have done your best to make others better, you should feel good with the warmth and contentment that will comfort you as the end nears. Do not dwell on what is next in your life, but, instead, laugh and smile as you revisit pleasant memories with your loved ones and friends. Celebrate your life and all the positive things that happened while you were involved. Your next journey is not to be feared. You will be in a better place."

This is what Marjorie had discussed with Thomas. It seemed to work most of the time, but there were times when the good doctor looked sad and was much quieter than normal. Nate actually carried the conversation during these times; he did quite well at it. One day he made mention of a lesson that Marjorie had taught him. As Thomas asked Nate several questions about the lesson, Nate noticed that the doctor's face went from sad to happy.

From then on Nate would revisit lessons from Marjorie whenever he saw distress in Thomas' face. He never wanted this kind man, his mentor and so much more, to suffer. He would do whatever in his power to alleviate any sadness in Thomas and for that matter, Marjorie as well. He had many wonderful lessons to revisit.

One day after work, Marjorie said that she had something for Nate in the house. When they arrived in the house, this wonderful baker of cookies gave Nate two of his favorite ones along with a big glass of water. She told him to sit, relax because he had done such great work, and enjoy the snack.

Nate said, "Thank you, I say yes to the first thing and, absolutely yes to the last thing. In addition," he smiled, touched Marjorie's shoulder, and said, "I only do great work because I have a wonderful teacher."

"Why thank you, Nate, for the compliment," a smiling Marjorie responded. She had noticed her prized student was giving her quite a few compliments in the last year. Not only were they greatly appreciated, but also it made her stop and think how far her wonderful boy had come. As Nate devoured the cookies and refreshed himself with the water, Marjorie started to think that maybe it was time for another tea with Mary. Yes, most definitely, M would arrange it fairly soon. The M girls never got tired of sharing stories about their son. Mary had told Marjorie that when they met for tea it would be perfectly fine for both of them to refer to Nate as our son. Mary explained to me that she deserved to use that special word, and Mary loved saying our son.

When Nate was finished with his snack, Marjorie told him that she had a letter for him, a long one. She explained, "It might take a couple of days to read and review the topics because it's important that you really think about the words. You can keep the letter; it is yours. You may write back if you like, but it is not necessary. At no time will I discuss the letter with you. We will converse about this letter only in writing. Is this okay with you?" She asked as she touched Nate's shoulder.

"Well, okay," replied Nate, "but I like asking my mentor and second mom questions with my oral communication skills." He smiled.

Marjorie's eyes watered up, and she spoke after a slight pause, "Thank you for those words. I love you like a son. Your mom said that I could say that to you; I've been wanting to for a long time." She hugged him for an extended time and kissed him on the cheek.

Nate managed to whisper, "I love you too."

When both individuals regained their composure to a degree, Marjorie handed the letter to Nate with the words, "I hope you enjoy it. It is meant to give you some information that you might use. You don't have to use any part of it, but just in case you need it, you will have it in writing to review. Of course, with your memory, you probably won't forget a word."

THE LETTER

This letter is strictly for you, Nate. It is my thoughts and opinions on growing up. It is probably not scientifically sound, or it is maybe not as accurate as one might like, so let us just keep it between us, okay? I believe there are three areas of growth that we humans go through. Physical growth is perhaps the easiest. As long as we take care of ourselves in a number of ways, we will grow into mature physical bodies. I have had the pleasure of seeing this transformation in you ever since you were two. Your parents did a marvelous job guiding your physical growth. You have become an amazing young man – tall, handsome, and strong. Again, thank your parents, but also thank yourself. You contributed so much in your physical journey to manhood. You have learned to work hard physically without damaging your body. The good habits you follow will benefit you for a lifetime. You should be so proud but don't ever forget the care your wonderful parents provided.

Skills and intellectual growth are more difficult to attain. Somewhere along the line to adulthood, a child will need mentors, people who provide lessons and skills training, to prepare them for work as an adult. Not every child benefits from good mentoring. Nate, you have had some of the very best mentors any child could ask for. I won't name them, but will say that it was my joy to be part of your education. It was a pleasure to watch you grow into adulthood with so many fine work skills, great social skills, along with a wonderful advanced intellect. All of your mentors love the man you have become. Most of all, your mentors love your propensity for kindness and concern for others. I truly believe these two things will lead you to something very special.

You should be so proud of the man you have become. Always remember your mentors provided the information, but you did the work. Be proud of that. Carry your skills and intellect as indispensable tools but never in a boastful manner. I know you would never do that, but it is something a teacher must say. You are too kind and respectful to brag. None of your mentors is boastful for very good reasons.

Intellectual and skills growth never stops. They will, very likely, get more refined, and along the way, wisdom will become part of your knowledge base. This gift of wisdom is usually based on life experiences and is usually refined by one's intellect. All of these things will grow to be quite sophisticated. I know that all your mentors would love to be there to see you display your intellect, skills, and wisdom later in your life. We all would be so proud.

Never forget what type of people your mentors were. This will help you if you get the chance to mentor someone in your future. I truly hope, if you get the chance, that you will become a mentor. It gives you a chance to help someone, support them in their learning, and guide them to success. It is one of the most rewarding things I have ever done. Of course, I had the most amazing student, maybe you have heard of him, Nate Johnson. (Smile)

Before I get involved in the third area of growth, I want to mention your parents again.

THEY ARE SIMPLY AMAZING! They have been there every step of the way and assisted you in all ways possible. I know you are going to do great things because you have modeled your life values very much like your parents. So many of your attributes are perfectly aligned with your folks. This makes me so proud of you. As you travel through life's journey, you are going to make so many people happy to have known you. Your good deeds, affinity for kindness and thoughtfulness, along with the extraordinary work you do, will make you a tremendous asset to any community to which you are part.

The third area of growth is, by far, the most complicated. It is very hard for me to write it down in an organized fashion, but I will try. At a young age, we start to become social beings with emotions. When we are young, the interaction is primarily with the immediate family. Your parents did a marvelous job. I saw some of the care, love, and support they provided for you. You were well taken care of.

Thomas and I became part of your life in a more formal setting when you were eleven years old. We had always enjoyed our visits, but this new situation involved formal teaching in several areas. The schooling was mentioned in the previous two areas of growth, so I will focus on teaching the social aspects of life. These aspects along with emotions are intertwined in our interactions with others.

Thomas' job was to teach by example. We both knew that you would learn so much by watching and listening to him as you two went through your days together. Your intelligence and power of observation benefitted your learning tremendously. Always be proud that these things guided you to write down many great things in your journals. Thomas and I talked every day about what you learned that particular day. We were so happy during these discussions. We felt like parents.

My job was to teach you about the garden and some school topics. More importantly, I would demonstrate the social skills that we knew you would observe, write down, and eventually display yourself. Any appropriate social skills that your mother and I deemed necessary at that particular time would be added to my list of skills to teach. Yes, your mother and I talked periodically about your social skills and what we could do to enhance them. This is one reason why your mother and I are so close. In fact, I want to share a story with you. Your mother is involved, but I don't think she would mind. She will never know anyway. Right? (Smile)

When you were about fourteen years old, we had been working together for nearly three years, and I realized that I had developed an emotional bond for you that might have been more than a mentor should establish with a pupil. I was not sure what to do. I liked the emotion; it made me happy inside. It gave me warmth. I did not want to stop this emotion, but I thought maybe I should. I needed guidance. I will talk to the minister – no – I will talk to the minister's wife. (Joke) I hoped you smiled.

One day when you were going to be working with your dad, I invited your mother over for tea. I was apprehensive and somewhat nervous, but the topic needed to be discussed. I explained the situation and apologized, along with saying that it just rather happened. I explained that I would step back over time to reestablish a proper mentor/student relationship.

Nate, your mother started to cry. My eyes watered up. I thought I would really hurt your mom's feelings. Then she asked me if she could give me a hug. Your mother went on to explain that three years ago she told your father that she would be willing to share her son with me. On that day of our first memorable tea, she told me that it was okay for me to love her son. She was sure that her son loved me.

Then your mother added, "Who wouldn't love the most amazing lady I've ever met?" Nate, of course, I had my handkerchief out as your mother went on to say that it has been an extreme pleasure sharing her son and discussing his lessons and progress for the past three years. Then she added, "We make a good team."

I am going to start social interactions with something I personally know will never happen or take place with you. SALOONS they are generally a bad place, in my opinion. Alcohol and good manners do not always go well together. If you throw in gambling, things get worse. Many times, language gets rough and tempers come to the surface. I have never been in a saloon. Thomas has been in a few for a very short time in the afternoon. Stay away from saloons completely in the evening. Behavior is much worse then. I have asked around, and many wonderful people have never entered a saloon.

Why did I mention saloons? It is simply that as we grow into adulthood, we must learn to interact with people. It is a highly refined skill. You very likely will never hear this refinement demonstrated in a saloon. People die because of actions that take place in a saloon. Always beware.

Your mother and I are extremely proud of your highly developed social skills. You are respectful, well thought out, a great listener, and never boastful. You enjoy talking with all types of people, oftentimes using humor that goes so well with your charm. You have learned to give smiles and compliments to people. These are such powerful and positive things. Continue to use them to benefit so many. You have learned to laugh easily but never at someone, good for you. We are so proud. You should be too.

You will continue to develop these skills, as you get older. It gets easier because you build on what you already know. Nate, you have the skills to venture out into the world on your own. Your five mentors all agree with this assessment. Of course, you would never leave us at this moment, but things can change. If they do, you will be prepared.

In the last five years, your mother and I have seen your emotional life develop nicely. You display your affection to others with your hugs, smiles, touches, and laughs. It has been a wonderful thing to watch. We truly believe you are ready for the next step, a relationship with a young woman. We know that you do not really know anyone at this time, but there may come a time when someone might appear in your life. This person might catch your fancy. Your mother and I want you to know that you have all the skills necessary to pursue a relationship. Will you be nervous? Yes, most young men are. Please remember that the young woman will, very likely, be nervous also. Thomas could barely talk the first time we met, and we turned out just fine. Just be yourself and be honest.

Like every good teacher, I should summarize and review my lesson. Your physical growth is just about over. You have become a tall, muscular; handsome young man, be proud but never boastful. Your intellect and skills are well above average. Your mentors are so proud. Continue to refine your skills as you travel through the years. You will make a fine mentor one day. Your greatest achievement to date has been your social interaction with everyone you encounter; it is marvelous to see. I have seen you teaching your brother and sister different things. You are knowledgeable, personable with many smiles and laughs, and demonstrate a wonderful emotional interaction with them both. TRULY

HEARTWARMING I truly hope that as you travel down life's road you will share: your skills, laughs and smiles (so important in life); knowledge and insight, friendship (one word, but so critical in life); and last, but not least, love. You have so much to give. I love you.

Nate wrote a short note to Marjorie that thanked her several times. He really enjoyed writing it and knew his primary mentor would like reading it. He smiled at that thought.

I always enjoyed being taught by my mentors. It was a joy to learn so much, but my greatest joy was you. You taught me about life. I now love to laugh, smile, and feel emotion. Thank you for teaching me these things. They help me to give just the right type of compliments, which I love giving. I love to make people smile and feel good. Thank you for showing me so many smiles over the years and giving me such wonderful compliments. As I journey forth into the world giving as many smiles and compliments as possible, I will often think of your words, smiles, and love that you had for me. Experiencing these things taught me to enjoy loving you.

At a town gathering when I was eleven, you took my hands and told me you would help me with any questions that I might have. You smiled and held my hands. I didn't understand it at that time, but I do now. I started to love you at that moment. You taught me about feelings. I now openly tell my family that I love them. I also love your amazing husband. You taught me this. My life is so much more complete with love as part of it. Thank you for enriching my life. I want you to know that one day I hope to find the kind of love that you and Thomas share. All of these years with you have prepared me for my adult journey. My two mothers have been more than a blessing. I LOVE YOU!

A short time later, the Smiths went to see a heart specialist. Thomas knew what was going on, but he wanted advice as to what steps should be taken. Were there any medications that might be helpful? They would be gone five days. Nate would be in charge. It was the most responsibility he'd ever had. The Smiths had left for a period a couple of times before, but Thomas brought in a veterinarian to cover. Now, if an emergency popped up, it was going to be Nate to the rescue. His father offered to help. Nate thought that was kind, so much like his father. There was one birth, a small foal. Jeremy was as impressed as to how Nate handled everything. He praised him several times. Nate liked that as well as the fact Thomas had said any money you make would be yours. Nate was paid for being a vet.

When the Smiths came back to town, they had a Negro woman with them. Thomas explained later to Nate that the good woman had lost her cooking and cleaning job. Her boss had been an absolute tyrant. Marjorie saw Mabel sitting on some steps near where the Smiths were staying and asked if she was okay. The next thing you know Mabel was on the train heading home with the Smiths. This was so typical of them. When a neighbor needs help, you help. Another lesson Nate had seen before, but this was somewhat different. Mabel was a total stranger.

Nate found out very soon that Mabel was going to be living with the Smiths, doing the cooking, and cleaning. Marjorie would help some, but Mabel was a fine cook and would do the majority of the work. After thinking for a couple of days about what the Smiths had done for Mabel, Nate decided that helping a stranger is perhaps the highest level of giving. It demonstrates the utmost kindness and goodwill. Nate would remember this for the rest of his life.

Of course, Nate wondered what the heart specialist said; he never found out. It was not his business to ask. His father had taught Nate years ago that another individual's personal business was private. You should not ask questions because you might be butting in. If they want you to know something, they will initiate the conversation. He explained that this was an important lesson. He mentioned that he always has to be careful when talking to church members, so as not to pry where he is not wanted.

Nate ate most meals with the Smiths since he lived on the property. He was still so very thankful that Thomas had suggested building a small cabin style dwelling behind the Smiths' home. It was out near a stand of trees with great sun in the morning and cool shade in the afternoon. The kind doctor explained to his right hand man, "I've always wanted to build a small place out there. It would be the perfect location. We could use some of the trees for part of the cabin." He finished up by saying, "Your father, you, and I can build it. That sounds like so much fun for all three of us."

All Nate had said to Thomas was that he was thinking about possibly moving out, or, at least, building another room onto the Johnsons' place. Later, Nate figured that the Smiths had probably already discussed him coming to live on the property. It gave Nate some space, privacy, and some feeling of independence. Once again, he realized how special the Smiths had been in helping him.

His father, Andy, and Doris were in favor of the move, but Nate's mother was hesitant. She didn't say why and finally said okay on a trial basis. Building the cabin was so much fun. It took some time because they worked on it part time. Nate learned from both his dad and Thomas; they both knew quite a bit. Thomas and Jeremy became even better friends during the building. They shared laughs and smiles every time they were together. Nate really liked that. An example that Nate would never forget was the time that his father said to Thomas, "Can you give me a hand?"

Thomas replied, "I can't, I need it for my practice." Jeremy laughed, as did Nate. That was typical of the interaction between the three.

Mabel was indeed a fine cook. Thomas and Nate had to be careful not to overeat. Meals were very pleasant as all four at the table shared some stories of the present and past. Mabel shared the most. All three kept her busy with many questions. One thing was perfectly clear; Mabel enjoyed being part of the family. Marjorie had told her on the very first day when she moved in that she was family now. Each day the family grew closer together. The Smiths were amazing at making Mabel feel very comfortable.

It did not come as a big surprise that one night at dinner Jack Brown attended. Marjorie had asked Mabel if it would be okay to invite Jack. Nate thought there might have been an example of a recent lesson for him to witness. Jack was somewhat shy and at a loss for words at the beginning of dinner; Mabel was much quieter than normal. Luckily, the Smiths are champions at conversation, and soon everyone was at ease. It must have been a pleasant evening because the next week Nate was cooking dinner for the Smiths. Mabel was dining at Jack's.

Mary thought of Marjorie a number of times during most days. Especially after the Smiths' return from the specialist. Nate kept his mother informed of Marjorie's condition on a weekly basis. Mary wondered if their teas were outdated. She sure had enjoyed them. The closeness she felt with M was more than anything she had ever experienced. They were definitely kindred spirits, but it was even more than that. Mary was an only child. Maybe Marjorie was the big sister she never had. That might explain the strong bond and love that existed between the two women.

A short time later after the Smith's return, Mary received a note from M discussing getting together for tea, pastry, and great conversation. Marjorie mentioned Monday as the house was going to be empty for several hours. She suggested 10:30. Mabel will leave us some of her fantastic pastries. I have some new tea I would like you to try. Look forward to your visit. Signed M Mary had Andy run a response back to M immediately. It simply said, Monday, 10:30 a.m., sounds divine, signed M2. Mary was concerned as to how much crying she would do. She had no idea why M wanted to talk, but M2 knew it was important for her to go. She wanted to explain her sister theory no matter how much she cried.

At 10:30 sharp, Marjorie opened the door for her guest and the two women embraced for quite a while without a word being said. The emotion was too strong. Finally, Marjorie spoke, "I am so glad you could come over. I look forward to our visits in so many ways. I was talking to Nate a couple of days ago, and I was so happy with what he was saying that I immediately thought of you. So, let's have some tea as I explain."

They walked to the dining room table hand in hand. Upon reaching the table after walking fifteen steps without talking, Mary said, "What did our son say, M, that you want to share?"

M gently squeezed M2's hand, smiled, and said, "Thank you for saying 'our son'. I am always a little nervous to say it first. Have you been getting a lot of compliments from our son?"

Mary answered, "No, not any more than usual. He has been more talkative in the last year. He mostly talks about you."

Marjorie poured the tea after telling Mary to please sit. She explained that Mabel set the table. She has been a wonderful addition to our family. When you come to dinner this Saturday, she will be doing the cooking; she is very good. By the way, Jack will be joining us if that is okay with you.

M2 smiled and responded, "How wonderful. I will tell the family, but I know they will be thrilled. The kids all love Jack, and our son says Mabel is simply amazing.

Okay, my big sister, tell me what's on your mind."

M reached over and touched Mary's arm as she said. "M2, I really like that you just called me your big sister." She paused, and then went on. "Our son's been giving me many compliments. He has gotten good at it. Thomas says he is getting them too. Nate seems so comfortable, always smiling, with words just coming out quite animated. It is so splendid to experience. I just had to tell you that I believe our job may be done. We have taken our little boy and made him into a fantastic man. I just had to share this with you." Mary took Marjorie's hand into both of hers and said, "I have been kind of thinking the same thing and have wanted to tell you. Our son is a wonderful, caring, and immensely talented young man. He has taken what you and Thomas have taught him and used it to learn new things. It is so much more than enjoyable to see. Doris and Andy are actively learning from their older brother; I just love it. Our job with Nate is done. Changing subjects, I want to say something that may be a touchy topic."

"Our son's role at your house has changed. He is bright and knows what is going on. He wants to comfort you and Thomas. One day he and I talked about it. He said that when he was young, the Smiths always comforted him at town gatherings. Now that he has learned from you two to be more social, he really wants to be a comfort for both of you. It was his idea to compliment, smile, and make jokes the best he could. He said it was easy with both of you because you each smile and laugh so readily when the three of you are together. Many of his social mannerisms duplicate what he saw in you and Thomas. The two of you have given him your incredible people skills, and I love you both for it.

"Nate loves both of you, but his feelings and my feelings for you are beyond special. I could not figure out or explain my feelings for you. I am an only child. My only way to explain the bond I feel for you, the love I hold in my heart, and the abundance of pleasant memories I have stored away is to make you my big sister who helped me raise my young son. You will travel with me, by my side, for the rest of my life. I will fondly remember our sister teas. I will talk to you, explaining what is happening with the Johnson clan. I will remember our smiles and laughs. I will laugh and smile again as I remember your words. I will always love you and will, from time to time, cry tears of joy as I am doing now for having you in my life. I know that one day we will be together again."

Marjorie walked over next to Mary, took her hands in hers, lifted them slightly so that Mary would rise up, and gave her a strong hug saying, "M2, I've always wanted a little sister."

Chapter 8

A Sad Time

Marjorie and Mary met often in the six months following their epic tea where Mary had explained to me that she thought of her as a big sister. With Doris and Andy so much older, M2 felt that they could be completely left on their own. She had more free time and why not spend it with her "sister".

On the third drop by visit, Mary initiated the hug with the words, "Hello, big sister." She also gave her a kiss on the cheek. Mary did not care if Mabel saw or heard.

Of course, M responded with the words, "Hello, little sister." She in turn gave Mary a kiss on the cheek.

They laughed as they told stories of the past. Both shared information that sisters would talk about; things nobody else knew. They did not talk about the inevitable. On the first drop by visit, M had given Mary the letter for Nate about Abigail's last lesson. She wanted her approval, but, more importantly, she wanted Mary to understand and follow the lesson. Both understood that it would dictate the foundation of their future visits. Mary gave me some of her private poetry. They enjoyed talking about the poetry; Mary was a big fan. Mary had never shown it to anyone before but felt Marjorie would enjoy it and appreciate the topics.

One day Mabel answered the door and explained that Marjorie wasn't up yet. There was a look of concern on Mabel's face. Mary thanked her for the information and explained that she would be discreet. As she walked home, she knew the time was coming. She kept saying to herself the whole way home, "I was so lucky to have her in my life." She still cried some.

Thomas stopped going on calls except for Tuesday and Friday afternoons. Nate covered all the other times. On the afternoons when Thomas did go out, Nate was in the house with Marjorie. He also dropped in every morning to say hello if Marjorie was up. He was still able to make his second mom smile, and she loved his visits. One afternoon Marjorie told Nate that she wanted to sit by the window and feel the warm sunlight.

Nate said, "Today I will call you 'Sunshine' several times as I see the sun brightening your beautiful face. Sunshine also reminds me of the thousands of smiles you have given me that brought sunshine into my heart."

Marjorie said, "That's a wonderful thing to say, my dear son. Thank you, it certainly brings back so many fantastic times that we have shared. Can I have a hug?"

"Well, you certainly can," replied a smiling Nate. "You can have two. I'm having a special on them today." They embraced for quite a while. She didn't get up; Nate leaned in from the left, kissed her twice along with saying, "I love you, Mom" twice. He finished up by saying, "I'm having many specials today, Sunshine. Teacher, do I capitalize sunshine when I say it?" Marjorie smiled and squeezed his hand.

"You certainly make our visits so very special. I think of them for hours after you leave. Sometimes I share them with Thomas. He enjoys hearing about our visits. Now tell me about your last few days of work. Tell me everything," said a smiling Marjorie.

Nate always tried to do most of the talking, as he knew Marjorie's energy level was down. He reviewed his work over the last two days and then quickly started reminiscing about all the wonderful times they had shared. Nate loved this part of the visit, as did M. He made Marjorie smile and laugh as he reviewed past lessons. He thanked her numerous times for helping him to become the man he is today. He hugged her and kissed her cheek often. It was now his turn to help her.

As Nate left for his cabin after a touching visit with M, he really appreciated what his mother had told him when he was eighteen.

"Your father has a great speaking voice; people love listening to it. My talented son has the same voice. Don't be afraid to use it. Everyone will enjoy it." As Nate continued his thoughts, he knew that M did seem to like his voice. This gave Nate more confidence in speaking than he'd ever had before. He started to think his voice just might be another "tool" he could use.

The dinners continued until near the end. Mary told Doris and Andy to explain to the

Smith is how school was going along with any interesting chore stories. She explained the Smiths love a good story. The Smiths stayed on the porch before and after every dinner listening to the Johnsons expound about their lives. The Johnsons always included several thank you to the Smiths for what they had done for the family. The Smiths loved it, as did all the Johnsons. Mary had done a good job preparing everyone.

Then one day she was gone.

That day when Nate got home from work, he saw Thomas and Mabel sitting on the steps of the porch. He knew. He ran to get his mother. Marjorie and Mary planned this out several weeks before. M2 had a letter for Thomas to be read by Jeremy at the Johnson's house when the time was right. Marjorie and Mary had written it sometime before. The Johnsons were to keep Thomas overnight at their home after the letter was read. Nate would contact the necessary people. Mabel had already changed Marjorie into her favorite dress that morning with M's help. Mabel told Mary the next day that Marjorie knew it was her last day. She had told Mabel to give Thomas a small snack and send him to their room. They were not to be disturbed but please comfort him when he comes out.

Jeremy was home when Nate came running in. The buggy was ready to go per Mary's instructions. M and M2 had talked briefly two days ago. They had already planned everything, but Mary loved going over to visit. M2 would hold her sister's hand as she told Marjorie stories about when they first met. Mary made it entertaining. She smiled, squeezed M's hand when she came to special parts in the story, and asked Marjorie certain questions like, "Do you remember the time you gave Doris that beautiful doll?" These types of questions elicited a short response and always a smile from M. Mary would then expound on the topic to M's delight. M2 was quite good at this style of conversation. She had used this same format in her years of teaching, so everything was smooth and comfortable. M2 loved it. It felt very fulfilling for Mary to bring joy to her sister. Every once in a while, M2 would lean in for a hug and a kiss on the cheek. She always added a few comforting words. M enjoyed this and told M2 how special her visits always were. At the end of the visit, Marjorie told Mary that her time was just about over, three days at the most.

Jeremy, Nate, and Mary rode the buggy to the Smiths' house. Mabel had been briefed on what was to happen. She was to take the buggy to Jack's place, and when they were ready, they would come to the Johnsons' for dinner. Nate would walk into town to do his part. Everybody he was to see had been briefed as to what to do. Mary and Jeremy would walk Thomas back to the Johnson house where Jeremy would read the letter. Mary had done most of the planning and even wrote the letter with some help from M. She loved doing it because of all the things her big sister had done for her and Nate. She told Marjorie on the last visit that helping was the least she could do for the best big sister in the world.

Jeremy read the letter on the porch as soon as the three got back to the house. He had a gift in the way he spoke at these times. Mary did not know how he did it. Maybe it was the number of times he had done it, but he was very comforting.

MARJORIE'S LETTER TO THOMAS

My dearest Thomas, we have had some wonderful talks in the last year where we shared some life-endearing thoughts and heartfelt emotions. I enjoyed them so much. They were intimate and amazing, and I hope they have helped prepare you for your continued journey with your many friends and family. Most people do not know how strong you are, but I do. When your parents died several years ago, you showed great strength. My dear Thomas, we talked often, and you were able to keep them in your heart and on your mind, but you returned to a normal life rather quickly. Many people were impressed, myself included. People have always said that Dr. Smith has a great sense of humor, a wonderful contagious smile, and a gift of words. You need to share these wonderful traits as much as you can. I know that in the past, we have always been there to comfort and support each other, but you are a member of the Johnson and Brown families now. All members are there to comfort and support you. Talk and be active. Enjoy Nate. Take great pleasure in what you helped create. Work with wood with Jeremy. He would enjoy that. Sing with Jack and Mabel. You have always loved their singing. If you get a chance, spend some time with my little sister, M2; she is the most marvelous woman. You will enjoy the conversations; I guarantee. Befriend Doris and Andy like any good uncle would. Buy them some gifts from time to time and make something for them with your creative wood skills. Learn as much as you can about them. They, along with Nate, are the future of the Johnson family of which we are part. Mentor them all.

Shortly later, Jack and Mabel pulled up in the buggy. Thomas was with Doris and Andy, who were asking him questions along with explaining what they do. Mary had, of course, arranged this. From a distance, she could see that Thomas wasn't himself, but he was interacting with the children. Baby steps were needed at this time. Keep him busy until the shock calms down. Nate joined the group in the garden and gave Thomas a rare hug along with the words, "I love you, my mentor." Thomas smiled and nodded but didn't say anything. Nate thought that was okay. Like his mother, he knew it would take countless little steps to move Thomas back towards normal.

The young handsome and intelligent man also knew his veterinarian mentor would never be the same. That would be impossible. Part of what Thomas was involved Marjorie being by his side. She made him better; he made her better. The loss created a void that couldn't be filled. The whole town wouldn't be the same. Nate had also been struck hard by the event of the day. He wondered if he would ever be the same. Marjorie had taught Nate about Abigail's resilience. M's brilliant mother always returned to doing good deeds and being a positive influence after she had experienced tragedy. Giving kindness, smiles, and compliments were just part of who Abigail was. Maybe Nate should concentrate on demonstrating all the lessons M had taught him. He had used them extensively when comforting Thomas and Marjorie recently. It was very pleasurable using the smile, small talk, and compliment lessons. They were definitely a positive influence; he liked that. Nate decided that he would move forward by using M's lessons.

That night Doris, Andy, and Nate slept in the Johnson's small barn. They had moved the buggy out to make room. To everyone's surprise, Thomas slept there too. He and Nate talked well into the night. Thomas explained that he was not sure he could go home. He explained that he had gone into the house after sitting with Mabel on the porch. The grief he felt was overwhelming. Mabel had to hold him and talk to him for a long time to calm him down. He didn't want to experience that emotion again. He asked Nate if he could sleep in the cabin with Nate taking the house. That was agreed upon, along with the fact that the kind doctor wanted Mabel to stay on. He asked about the arrangements, and Nate explained that it was all taken care of per Marjorie's wishes. He informed Thomas of the details.

The next morning after breakfast, Thomas, Nate, and Mary walked back to the Smiths' house. Mabel was there cleaning the house. She heard them talking as they walked up and went outside to greet them. Thomas smiled, gave her a hug, and said, "Good morning Mabel, thank you for your help yesterday. I don't know what I would have done without you."

Mabel kissed him on the cheek and responded, "You have been so kind to me. I just had to help you on such a sad occasion. It is what you do with family. I am so sorry. If Jack and I can do anything, please let us know."

Mabel excused herself and went back inside to finish cleaning. Thomas asked Nate and Mary to come and sit on the porch. "I feel her here today," Thomas said. "I think she wants me to share something with both of you. Mary, you might benefit from what I say as you're speaking at the funeral." Marjorie loved this town. She explained to me over the years that this town was our home and the people in it were our extended family. She loved working and helping wherever she could. It gave her great pleasure. She never wanted to travel because she had everything right here that she ever wanted or needed. Mary, M said that you know who to place as her one thing that made her feel complete.

"At a town gathering years ago, Marjorie and I befriended a little boy named Nate that led to the greatest ten years of our lives. We were able to become members of the Johnson family. Both of us grew to love the Johnson clan. Marjorie developed a bond with Mary that led them to become sisters. It was such a fantastic relationship. Words cannot describe the love and closeness between you two amazing women. Mary, you are so very special. Above all, we cherished our time with Nate. We were able to see his growth as we helped him develop through the years. Every evening we talked about 'our boy'. It made us feel like parents. We also felt a wonderful connection to Jeremy, Doris, and Andy, much like blood relatives."

"M felt so much love here in this town. It filled her heart, and every day was a joy. Therefore, Mary, tell the dear town members not to grieve for her. She has been blessed during her life in this town. Encourage them to please continue to do good deeds and be kind. Marjorie will smile when she sees those things. You all know that she will be watching from above. She wants everyone to know that she has been blessed to have lived a life well lived. She loves you all."

Thomas asked Nate to tend to the garden, as he would like to talk with his mother privately. He then explained to Mary that for many years Marjorie had no family left. By the time she was thirty-five years old, her family was gone. She had seen quite a bit of tragedy.

It took a very long time for her to be able to talk about her mother without tearing up.

Marjorie was not a person to be mired in self-pity, another lesson from her mother. Everybody loved her mother; M was so much like her. The loss of her nephew was also difficult to overcome but for a different reason. He was much like your Nate and M thought she was the one person who could help her sister's son, but she never got a chance.

Thomas continued to speak, "Many friends called her M when she was younger. She loved that nickname. After we moved here, she told me that she only wanted her wonderful husband to call her that. She did not want to get too close to people, as it had been so painful to lose some of her friends. Marjorie's brother and sister had also disappeared from M's life. She decided to focus on doing good deeds, being a positive influence, and loving her Thomas."

"Then you came along. She grew to love you and then you called her M, followed by lighting up her heart even more by whispering big sister during a hug. She truly felt that she had someone again, a person like her mother, who she had worshiped. Your relationship with my wife during these last several years has been way beyond special. The things you two shared, the help you provided, and your care and assistance created a deep family love. Mary, you probably know that Marjorie was extremely wealthy, close to a million dollars. My family left me more money than I will ever spend. Marjorie made me promise to make you take some money because you are her sister. She knows you will say no, but I will not accept that answer. The money is for the Johnsons. Use it for schooling for Doris and Andy. Keep some for a rainy day along with the idea that it is nice to have a stash. Marjorie hopes that when you think of the money, you will think of her. She would like that."

"Nate will be taken care of later. M did not want to influence his work ethic. He should learn to work over time to create some valuable assets and some rainy day money. It is important when you are young to learn to work for your money. She did not think money would change Nate but did not want to chance it. M hopes that one day he will do great things with the money that will be left to him. Please say yes to my request. I do believe Marjorie is here. It would please her immensely if you took the money."

It was hard for Mary to speak. The Johnsons were not poor by any means, but they never had extra. Yes, they did have a small stash. It was nice to have, a feeling of security. Now this wonderful woman, my sister, wants to help. "Thomas, I did know Marjorie was wealthy, but I didn't ever befriend her in order to receive money. I started to love her for her help with Nate. The rest just grew out of a true love for Marjorie as a person. You must know how easy it is to love her."

Thomas quickly responded, "I do, oh, how so much I do. M told me this last year that you two are so much alike: smart, honest, kind, and personable. Each of you has a smile that makes people smile right back. This is why she thought you two were sisters. M loved every part of you. She knew you would reject the offer. It is a very small amount of her wealth. By the way, her daddy earned the money in an evil fashion, and Marjorie wanted to do good things with as much of it as she could. Your taking the money would be a good thing, and it might help you. Marjorie would be so happy to help. Besides that's what sisters do. Right?"

"This is so generous. I will say yes, depending on what Jeremy says. I think he will agree. Doris and Andy are strong students. They both want schooling past what we have to offer here. The money would definitely help. Thank you so much, Thomas. I am going to walk away now to talk to my big sister. I told her six months ago that I will always carry her by my side and will talk to her often," replied a teary-eyed M2.

Mary did walk away towards home after giving Thomas a hug. She squeezed his hand as she turned and walked away. She had seen Nate heading towards them and did not want him to see any tears. She had some editing to do on her eulogy, as she wanted to make it as perfect as possible. Jeremy was going to stand beside her to step in if Mary needed a few seconds to regroup. He knew the content of the speech and could step in without missing a step. The people in attendance would think it was planned. Jeremy had volunteered to do this because he knew how important it was to Mary for the delivery to be as smooth as possible.

When Nate arrived at Thomas' side, he suggested to his mentor that they work on a small addition to his cabin. He brought some paper to write down some measurements and a list of materials that would be needed. Thomas asked Nate what was needed in the cabin. He thought the place was complete. Nate explained that a small kitchen with three windows would be a splendid addition. He said that he would pay for all the materials. Thomas said that he appreciated the offer, but he would pay for everything because that is what Marjorie would want. He asked Nate if he could feel her presence. Marjorie's son said only one word, "Yes."

Thomas smiled, touched Nate's shoulder much like Marjorie would have done, and stated, "I'm so glad you feel her here today. There are three people in a world that M will have trouble-saying goodbye to. I think she will leave when she knows we are all okay. It is impossible to put into words the love she felt for you, but you probably already knew that. Every lesson she taught you was a labor of love. The more you grew, the happier she became. She and your mother's friendship grew into a big sister-little sister relationship. The love between these two was a rare thing to find. I think it made both of them so happy. This would not have happened if we hadn't become mentors to you."

"I truly believe that Marjorie was an angel sent to earth to do good things. I also believe that you are a major part of her mission. You will use all the things M taught you to do good deeds and be a positive influence in people's lives. Now, back to your cabin, or should I say my cabin since I will be sleeping there for a while. We are going to need your father, as he is the best finish carpenter of the three of us. You ask him sometime today, and we'll get started right after the ceremony."

The funeral was very well done, from the flowers to the music, the words from Jeremy, and a beautiful eulogy from M's sister. It was personable with some stories about the town that everyone enjoyed. Mary made everyone laugh several times. She smiled often and focused on how lucky we all were to have known Marjorie and be the recipients of her friendship, good deeds, and that wonderful smile. Jeremy had to step in here for a moment and he did it so smoothly that no one knew. Mary had given him a signal by squeezing his hand. He told the story about having dinner at the Smiths for the first time. He made it funny and even Thomas laughed. Mabel and Jack sang several songs.

There were no sad songs, just fun and upbeat songs. Jeremy had told the gathering earlier that Marjorie did not want sad songs. This was not to be a sad occasion, just a goodbye among friends until we meet again. It all went so well. Mary was relieved that it was over, but she knew that her big sister would have nothing but glowing words about the ceremony. This made Mary so proud of what she had orchestrated and pleased that the ceremony was very much like one Marjorie would have planned. Mary couldn't help but think that it was like M and M2 together for one last time.

Marjorie wanted a town gathering after the service with lots of food and plenty of music. Mary had hired a professional band. They were great. It didn't take long for the town to thoroughly enjoy the evening. M would have enjoyed the outing completely. When Thomas was dancing with Doris and then with Mary, he felt a warmth from within. He wasn't sure at first, but he then realized that M was giving her approval.

The next day was Sunday, and Thomas spent the whole day with the Browns and Johnsons. First, it was breakfast at the Johnsons' place, followed by church, and back to the Johnson's. The Johnsons changed into work clothes, and the group then walked to the cabin where Thomas changed. It was decided by Jeremy that some activity on the new addition wasn't work. It was going to be fun. Jack and Mabel joined them. As the eight people "played" around the cabin, the singing started and was enjoyed by all. Jeremy taught Andy some things about building, and Mary explained to Doris about the footing and preparing the ground. After an hour, the women left to prepare lunch. It was a splendid day, topped off by the announcement from Jack and Mabel that they were going to get married.

Thomas slept in the cabin; Nate occupied the house. The next morning after breakfast, Thomas told Nate he wanted to visit a few customers who had approached him at church. He asked Nate to work in the garden as it looked like it needed some work. He said he would see Nate for lunch somewhere around 1p.m.

Thomas arrived at 12:55 and didn't look good. Nate knew he had been crying. What could the student do to help his wonderful mentor? "Are you okay?" asked Nate.

Thomas replied, "No, I've had a rough morning. It is difficult seeing the many things in town that M and I helped build. They used to bring joy, but now everything has changed. Several women turned away when I approached because, I believe, they were starting to cry. A couple of people treated me very differently. They were nervous as to what to say. The only ones who seemed to enjoy my company were the animals." He smiled and went on, "Maybe I should buy some goats." He smiled again.

Nate said, "I am so sorry. Thomas, it will get better. People love your friendship and value your work. They will soon be back to a reasonable normal. Can I show you my work in the garden? I've been busy all morning. Mabel made me stop for some water at 11:00. This may be wrong to say, and I am sorry if it is, but I talked to Marjorie all morning. It made the time fly by, and I enjoyed it. Maybe you could try the same thing."

Thomas touched Nate's shoulder as he started walking toward the garden, and then he addressed Nate's comments, "Nate, thank you for the advice. It really sounds good. I have talked to Marjorie from time to time. It has not helped yet, but maybe it will in the near future. The garden looks great. Thank you for all the expert work. Now, let's have some lunch."

Thomas, Nate, Jeremy, and Andy built the addition. Jeremy really enjoyed having Andy there. When they were finished with the project, all agreed it was a great addition to the cabin. The three windows were perfect. Nate's design was quite good. His father said maybe he should be a builder like Jake. Nate enjoyed the compliment, and he really enjoyed the designing and building of the addition. Thomas and Jeremy talked constantly as they worked. Thomas didn't seem sad. Maybe the key was to keep his hands busy. It was a thought.

For the next three months, Nate and his mentor kept busy working together on many projects and vet business. One day the grown student asked his kind teacher, "Could I occasionally call Marjorie by her special name? I realize that it is a very special word. I don't want to interfere with that, but I know what Marjorie thought of the nickname. She felt the love and affection when the word was used. If she is listening from time to time to our conversations, I would like her to hear that name from me. I have so much love and affection for my second mom."

Thomas explained, "M was Marjorie's nickname in high school and college; she loved the name. The people who called her M were so dear to her, and these friends adored

Marjorie. The name, M, represented the love and affection between friends. Upon arriving in this town, I was the only one who called her M. It was a very special word, and then, after one of their special teas, your mother said to my wife, as they were saying goodbye 'I love you, M'. Marjorie told me later the name felt so right, in so many ways, coming from your mother. I truly believe, my grown-up student, that Marjorie would absolutely love you calling her M."

Most people were somewhat back to normal. Nate was succeeding in practicing all the lessons he had learned. He became quite friendly. Nate really liked it when some people said that he reminded them of the old Thomas. Thomas, on the other hand, had days where he was still grief stricken. Nate tried a number of things, as did Mary and Jeremy. Mary told the others that the hole in Thomas' heart might never heal. This was why Thomas could not attend Mabel and Jack's wedding. He knew he would break down, and he did not want to ruin such a joyous occasion. Mary understood completely and made the perfect excuse for her sister's husband. Mary still cried from time to time as she talked to me about the family.

One day Thomas told Nate, "I'm going to visit an old acquaintance some distance away to the west. The man is a lawyer in a town twice as large as the one we live in. He lost his wife five years ago and thought we could share some stories. The lawyer actually knew Marjorie quite well from college. That is how I met him. He is a good person. I will be gone a week. I have every confidence that you will be able to handle everything, just like last time. I leave tomorrow. I will drop by your parents' place to say goodbye. I have already told Mabel. She will continue to cook for you in the mornings but will be leaving at noon. She and Jack want to host your family for dinner one day while I am gone. Isn't that great?"

"It is," said Nate. "Our families are growing quite close. Everybody enjoys everybody.

Thank you for your confidence in me. I'm sure you will have a great trip."

Thomas returned in seven days. Nate thought he looked great; his walk, posture, and his whole demeanor were better. Thomas explained that the town was quite nice with many stores, restaurants, and specialty shops. He said, "You could spend a couple of days going from place to place. Outside of town, the landscape is beautiful. My lawyer friend says the town is growing." The vet mentioned that he enjoyed many aspects of the visit. Then he dropped a bombshell when he said he was thinking of moving there.

"You would actually leave your town, all your friends, and so many who love you? "Asked Nate.

"This is the hardest decision I've ever made. I love so much about this town. I feel connected to the Johnsons and Browns. It is a bond that I will miss very much, but I'm sad here, and I'm not sad there," said the kind doctor.

In two weeks, Dr. Thomas Smith moved from his beloved town that he and his wife helped build. The town knew how catastrophic the loss had been for Thomas. Many people also felt a hole in their heart. They also knew that this wonderful mentor; this amazingly skilled man; this kind and considerate human being needed a new start in a new location.

Chapter 9

A New Start

Thomas and Nate wrote regularly. As soon as one received a letter, they would sit down and start to compose a response. Both men missed each other for so many reasons: the mentoring, work, laughs, and friendship. Nate still had his family, work, and the Browns. Thomas was not so lucky. The letters from his friends were all he had. Nate's letters were usually the longest; Thomas usually read them twice. They were well written and contained a fair amount of humor. He found out that Nate was working with Jake Collins and really enjoyed it. He had learned so much about construction.

Nate wasn't working with Jack any more. He said that it was probably because Mabel was doing so much around the house along with all the cooking. This freed up Jack to spend more time working. The Browns were a good pair. It was also pointed out that the newlyweds were expecting. Thomas was thrilled for Mabel and Jack in so many ways. Nate mentioned several times that this loving and talented couple adored the house, and they wanted to thank Thomas as often as possible for being so kind. The vet thought it was only fitting that these newlyweds introduced by Marjorie should benefit from the house she built. It was her idea to bring Mabel back to town. It was another one of M's good deeds that benefited so many. Mabel had written Thomas a letter previously thanking him for all that he and Marjorie had done. Her life was now a blessing. She promised that she and Jack would do good things together.

Thomas kept all the letters he received. There were dozens of them, but the ones he enjoyed most were the ones from Nate and Mary. He knew who was responsible for the many letters. M had been so right about M2; she was so special. She always added humor to her letters. Thomas still liked to laugh, and Mary always made him do it. Nate's letters were very detailed. He told stories about people. The ones about Jack and Mabel were his favorite parts of a letter. Nate explained that one day Mabel told him, "Jack is such a wonderful husband. He is so kind and caring. He shows his affection in so many ways. He even said that he would build me a giant pedestal but knew that I was afraid of heights. We laugh and have such a good time together. He loves me so much." She then said that she believes that she loves Jack even more than he loves her. These words always warmed Thomas' heart when he reread them.

The vet's letters were much shorter than his protégé's. They didn't contain much detail and didn't exhibit much of Thomas' wonderful sense of humor. He didn't mention any friends that he had made besides the lawyer who had invited him to town. Thomas also did not mention a garden, to the point that Nate thought there was a possibility that there wasn't one. There was not one word about his work with the local vet. This really troubled Nate because he knew how important this work was to Thomas. All of these things made Nate and his mother think that something was wrong. They agreed that this amazing man missed his friends and families. They were right; Thomas had not divulged that he was very lonely.

Thomas sometimes wondered why he had a gut feeling that he was supposed to be in this town. He couldn't explain it along with the fact that, at times, he felt Marjorie's presence. Maybe M wanted Thomas and Nate to be together one more time. One day he decided to invite Nate to come for a visit. The vet would sure enjoy the company. He had been missing Nate more than normal the last two weeks. Thomas had grown to realize how important Nate was to the Smiths. It was never mentioned, but for ten years, Nate was the focus of their attention. When Nate moved to the cabin behind the house, the closeness actually increased. Thomas also knew that Marjorie and Nate were completely connected. Nate was M's son. Helping to develop a child, who would accomplish more wonderful things, is one of the greatest achievements of a person's life. Marjorie and her lessons would live on in Nate. Thomas always remembered that Marjorie had been the one who suggested tutoring Nate. WHAT A BLESSING

Thomas wrote a letter asking Nate if he would like to come for a visit. He only hoped that Nate wasn't too busy. He even considered going back for a visit with everybody. The pain of losing M had subsided to a degree, and Thomas thought he might be able to go back.

He would wait for Nate's response before deciding anything. He received his reply from Nate six days after mailing his request. Nate was coming. He will be there on Wednesday. Thomas was thrilled.

When Nate arrived on the stagecoach, Thomas was there in his buggy. He had the biggest smile on his face. He didn't wait for Nate's customary handshake. He gave his "son" an extended hug. Thomas couldn't believe how great Nate looked. He was so tan. Nate explained working with Jake does that to a person. Before they went to Thomas' favorite restaurant for dinner, the vet said, "Thank you for coming to visit. I have missed my grown up student. Maybe you could teach me some things about building, now that you are a pro."

Nate replied, "I definitely could teach you how to hit your thumb with a hammer. I think I have done that about five times. Jake tells me it takes about ten times to learn not to hit your hand. I'm not looking forward to the next five."

Thomas laughed and responded, "I think hitting your thumb as a carpenter is part of the hazards of the job, but you are a quick learner. I will bet you will learn in five, isn't that great news? Confidence is the key. My dad used to say that if you think you might hit your thumb, you would. Just be confident that you will hit where you aim."

"Amazing," said the young carpenter, "I've been here two minutes, and you've already taught me something. I am going to have to get some journals and pencils immediately. It's great to have my mentor back." Thomas smiled.

Over dinner, the two men shared some great reminiscing; it was so good to visit in person. Of course, Nate had to ask about working with the local vet. Thomas explained, "The local vet, along with several other businessmen in town, value money over people. My lawyer friend told me to avoid these individuals. They can get tough when someone threatens their enterprises. I am now retired. This old laborer is looking to help some neighbors who might need some form of cheap labor." He laughed and said that he would pay someone to provide him with some good honest work.

Thomas finished this topic with a story about a rancher west of town, "The rancher and his sons are the local blacksmiths. There was another one in town, but he decided to move away. My lawyer friend says the rancher pushed the other "Smithy" out of town. Now the rancher can charge more for the work he and his sons provide for the town. You would not believe what I paid for horseshoes. They also provide much of the lumber for the town. My friend believes the storeowner works with the rancher to keep lumber prices high. It's an ugly mess and not fair to the hardworking people in the town."

"I often think of Marjorie and how she helped so many. Her good deeds and sense of community set the tone for our town. People followed her lead. The town people became kind and helpful; they enjoyed supporting their neighbors and being a positive influence. The town was full of smiles, nice compliments, and hearty laughter. Marjorie promoted these things wherever she went. I truly believe she would have been the same even if she were not rich. It's just who she was," said the retired vet...

Nate shook his head and said, "I don't understand how you could treat neighbors that way. Making money at your neighbor's expense is so wrong. How could you look people in the eyes? How could you sleep at night? I guess our town is special. Maybe you should move back. I would be a local hero if I brought you back. I've never been a hero before."

Thomas smiled, touched Nate's arm much like M used to do, and said that he had been thinking about that. He then explained to his "son" that the old town did not need him. There are so many caring people helping and supporting each other. The weekly farmers' market was a great idea from Marjorie that helped everybody. It brought everybody together. The local bank was M's idea. Marjorie funded the bank. No one knew this, so do not tell anyone. She told the banker to charge a very low rate, which he could keep. She explained that the bank's purpose was to help, not make money. If someone could not pay their loan, he was to talk to Marjorie. She said to the banker that at no time was he to threaten to take the farmer's land away.

Thomas also told Nate, "Maybe that's why I was drawn to this town. It is a challenge, but it is something that my dear M would have jumped right into. She always believed in doing good deeds and being a positive influence. This town could surely use some. I have met many people. Most are good hardworking Christian folks. Marjorie led the way in our town. She taught me so much. Maybe it's my turn to lead the way."

Nate was quiet for a few seconds. Thomas thought that maybe he had hurt his student's feelings by not moving back to his old town and family. He surely did not intend to do that. He quickly took Nate's hands and said, "Think about my words. You will understand my dilemma. I miss my town, but maybe I am needed here. I am very confused as to what to do, but there is one thing that I am positively sure of. I love the Browns and Johnsons, but most of all I love you."

Nate's response surprised Thomas, "Thank you for those words. I am so lucky because my love for you and M radiates throughout my body when I think about you two. Now, I completely understand your thoughts. M taught me so much about those same ideals. It makes me feel worthwhile when I help someone. I did a few vet visits before the new vet came to town. Several of the customers were struggling and didn't have anything to offer as payment. I quickly said that they could do me a favor somewhere down the line. You taught me that. Thank you so much for such a powerful lesson. As I left their place, I felt so good for helping someone in need. I now know how you felt the countless times you did the same thing."

Nate continued, "There's been a few times when I've helped Doris, Andy, or one of their friends with making or fixing something. I explained what to do next time to make it better. I felt like a mentor, what a tremendous feeling. I hope to be half as good at mentoring as you and M were to me. By the way, I continue to talk to M quite often. I am not sad any more when I do. I also talk to you. She and you are so much of who I am. Marjorie taught me about love. I will always love my family, but I especially love you and M. I am truly blessed to have my two biggest mentors by my side as I travel through life. I remember your lessons, I can talk to you when both I need to, and I have all your lessons to guide me down the road of life. I am very proud of the man I have become. I thank the Smiths every day for making this happen. If you and Marjorie need me to help you in your quest to benefit this town, please let me know."

Thomas was stunned. What was Nate saying? He did not think that his young protégé was saying he would move. He decided that a quick thank you would suffice at this time. Thomas wasn't sure that he could ask Nate to move to this town and leave his family. "Well, that's quite an offer, a wonderful one," said the smiling mentor. "Thank you very much. Let us think about it for a while and get back to it later. Let us move on to my little place and get you settled in. How does that sound?"

Nate replied, "Sounds great, but I'm serious about the offer. I have been thinking about my future lately. I like working with Jake, but it is not my calling. I like helping people, working with animals, and, unbelievably, working in the garden. I think I like that because that is where I talk to Marjorie so much. Mabel does not need my help, but she and Jack have offered some space next to my cabin. This is so kind of them; I have started breaking ground. Doris and Andy are busy with school and other activities, so I help in our family's garden, but that is the point. Something is missing. Maybe I need to get my own place."

As the two men climbed aboard the buggy, Thomas explained, "I somewhat know what you're talking about. When Marjorie and I were living with my parents after college, we both felt the urge to be on our own, even though we loved living with my parents. There was never any pressure from my parents to move, so we took our time and made the right choice. You are in a similar situation. You are blessed with two families that love you very much. Take your time. You will know when the right time comes along."

For the next two days, Nate and Thomas viewed the town and the surrounding countryside. The two thoroughly enjoyed each other's company. They laughed often, smiled, and discussed life in general.

An example of some of Thomas' words was, "Many times the choices we make as young men aren't necessarily right or wrong, but instead provide a direction or pathway to a particular vocation. Your father, for example, could have been a fine carpenter. He chose the ministry as his life's work, but he could have chosen a path involving wood. Both would have worked for him, but the town is so fortunate to have him at the front of the church on Sundays. He probably would have been a builder much like Jake. We both know how great he is. I was considering the law or veterinary medicine. Can you just see me arguing my case?" He smiled. "The advice I have is to take your time, pray on it, and follow your heart."

Nate really liked the local landscape. There was an abundance of trees and a nice lake fed by a small creek from some mountains nearby. Thomas explained that he loves going for a ride in the buggy a couple of times a week. He was even considering riding a horse on such trips. He hadn't ridden since he was single but used to enjoy it very much as a teenager. Nate informed his dear friend, "My father and I have ridden a couple of times lately. My mother was somewhat nervous at first but was assured that we would be safe." The vet told Nate that he had access to a couple of horses. The next day the two men were riding horses in the countryside.

While on the ride, the two spotted a rather large wagon hauling some lumber. Thomas informed Nate that this was the rancher he had mentioned earlier. He also threw in the fact that he did not like this man. Thomas explained that the rancher is the aggressive type. It is common knowledge that he cheated his neighbors over a loan to get their land, nothing illegal but not very honest or neighborly. He had three neighbors who needed some money after an unusual drought. The rancher loaned them some money with their ranches as collateral. He told everybody it was just a formality. He would never do anything hurtful to his friends. There had to be something of value to back up the loan; this was just good smart business. The rancher calmly said that he was smart and good at business, so it all made sense.

The day after the loan repayment was due; the rancher had the sheriff tell the people to vacate the land as they had failed to repay the loan in a proper fashion. He purposely waited one day after the loan was due to foreclose. He gave them no warning. The people were devastated. Thomas mentioned, "My lawyer friend knows all about this because he wrote the contracts, and the rancher insisted on the clause that he would get the ranch if the neighbor defaulted. He assured my friend that he would never foreclose on his neighbors. These people were his friends. Another reason I have a disdain for this person is that he is cruel to his horses. When I went out to the ranch on a call with the local vet, I saw the whip marks. I was so furious but couldn't say anything. I also noticed that there was no mention of payment. My friend tells me these two work in cahoots to keep the price of horseshoes up. I have more stories, but you get the point.

"The rancher is raising his sons to be the same type of businessman as he is. The wife, on the other hand, seems to be kind and caring, but she has no input on the running of the ranch. We go right past their ranch on the way back, so you will get a good look at the place. It's pretty amazing."

Nate didn't talk for a few minutes. Thomas didn't want to interrupt because he knew Nate was thinking. When Nate did speak, he only said that the rancher seems like an evil man. He explained that he couldn't talk because he was too angry. My father always preached not to talk in anger, so I will wait some before we talk about it. He then asked Thomas if there was a farmers' market.

Thomas explained that the storeowner also owns the building next door where all the homemade goods are sold. A farmers' market is not allowed within a mile of town. The town council passed this and you know who controls that. The rancher and storeowner make good money off the sales of the homemade goods. Nate stopped his horse, told Thomas to hold the reins, and ran off fifty yards where he screamed off and on for about five seconds. After calming down somewhat, Nate walked back.

"I have never been this upset in my entire life," exclaimed Nate. "What can be done?"

Thomas explained, "I have thought about some things, talked to a number of people including my lawyer friend, and helped to develop a tentative plan. Most of the ideas came from my friend. His name, by the way, is Dan Perkins, a very good person. I am only helping to fill in some gaps in a rather nifty plan. His idea would cost some money and would need a representative. If I decide to stay in this new town, I would take care of both needs." Thomas went on to point out that is why he was so divided between moving home versus helping this town. It is not an easy question to resolve.

Nate finally spoke, "I'm sorry about my outburst; I haven't done that since I was six. What the rancher, storeowner, and vet are doing is so wrong. They are purposely hurting their neighbors and friends. Maybe I shouldn't say friends because they probably don't have any friends except for the almighty dollar. They probably don't even like each other. I want to help."

Thomas thanked Nate and told him to talk to his parents. The mentor explained that he didn't think the three culprits were violent, but you never know. Dan is a fine lawyer and is still upset that the rancher actually took his neighbors' land. He helped them relocate. To this day, his eyes water up when talking about their fate. He even offered to pay off their debt, but the rancher wanted the land. The lawyer was helpless; the court ruled in the rancher's favor. Dan is committed to taking the crooks out of office and power. He knows so many people who can help.

Thomas said, "Our plan finishes with the residents voting for new town council members in three months. There are five council members, and we have five good men running, including Dan and myself. The plan includes the town paying for an outpost for the army. Dan knows the ranking officer. Colonel Jones has agreed to build the outpost if the town pays all costs. The army will purchase all the materials with my money. It won't be a large contingent of soldiers, just about twenty. There will be enough to patrol the area and keep the peace. The Colonel stated that the outpost would be beneficial to the soldiers as the current fort is too small. The army could launch patrols from the outpost and be in the area for any protection that might be needed."

"On every other Saturday, the outpost will host a town market. Once the soldiers are here, I will hire a young man to help me service the community's vet needs at a greatly reduced rate. The Colonel has agreed to have some army personnel work at the town market, not too many but enough to get the rancher's attention. The army will also frequent the town streets to keep a presence for all to see. I will hire a couple of Pinkerton types to monitor the rancher's movements. Dan knows a few people that do this type of work. Hopefully in three months, we'll have broken up this ring of thieves and given the town back to the people."

Nate smiled, touched Thomas' arm, and said, "Can I be the new vet helper?"

Thomas laughed and said, "Well, I can certainly vouch for your training. You'll need to go home and talk this over with your family. It is a big decision; they need to be included. I also want you to rethink this several times. You will also have to talk to Jake. I'll bet he wants to witness the five more whacks to your left thumb."

"My left thumb wants me to be a vet's helper," said a laughing Nate. "I will do as you ask my mentor. You should get an answer in two or three weeks."

The two men rode quietly for a time taking in the scenery. Both men had many thoughts swirling through their heads. As they neared the rancher's place, Thomas pointed out several of the superior parts of the ranch. It was quite special, well done in many ways. Nate was impressed and told Thomas that it was the best ranch he has ever seen. A short time later, the men turned in their horses and headed to town for a nice relaxing dinner.

That evening the two exchanged stories. Nate informed Thomas, "I've become someone somewhat special with troubled horses. There have been times when people asked me to come out and look at a horse who was not acting correctly. Sometimes I would take it back to Mabel and Jack's place for a couple of days. When the job was done, the people insisted on some type of payment even after I declined the offer. In the end, I would usually be paid. I couldn't believe that I was getting paid for doing something I love to do." The skilled worker mentioned, "When you and Marjorie paid me for working in the garden, I felt the same way. Getting paid for the work you love is totally amazing." Nate had noticed on his arrival that there was no garden. After thinking about it, he understood why. Thomas always spent his time in the garden with M. Life couldn't get any better than that. No M – no garden the smart young man did not bring up the topic; he knew better.

Thomas shared with Nate, "I am still grieving. Some days are still bad. It has been much better with you here. This is why I am considering moving back to our town. Maybe being with the people I love would help me overcome my grief, but I just can't get Me out of my mind when I'm there. I did meet a woman at church here. She seems nice, but I just don't know. She is pleasant to talk to. If you weren't leaving tomorrow morning, I'd have you meet her. She's about my age, widowed, with a nice smile."

The next morning the two intertwined men said goodbye at the town depot. Nate noticed a sadness in Thomas' eyes, and that is when he decided. "I'm going home to say goodbye to my family. It will take a couple of weeks to be back here permanently. I want to start a garden. You can help if you would like. I will also be looking for a job. Ask around for me if you get a chance. I'm very excited about my new start," said an upbeat Nate.

"I am thrilled with the news but remember don't put the cart before the horse. Talk to your family, take your time, and trust your heart," said the beaming vet.

At dinner two days later, Nate brought up the topic of moving. His father spoke first and explained, "Although this is a sad topic of conversation, it is not unexpected. We all realize that one day you might venture out on your own. We want you to know that you can stay here forever if you would like, or if you leave, you will always be welcomed home. You are well equipped to travel out on your own. We like the fact that Thomas will be nearby. We love you, son, and are extremely proud of the man you have become." With those words, Jeremy stood up, walked over to Nate, pulled him up, and gave him the biggest hug ever. All five members of the family had tears in their eyes with a few running down their cheeks every now and then.

Mary did not speak for a while as she wiped tears away. She finally spoke, "I knew this day would come because it's part of your continued growth that M and I planned for. No mother wants their children to leave home, especially one that brings so much love and kindness to the household. You have helped to teach your brother and sister those things, and because of it, we have such a wonderful family. I love it every day. I love M for helping to make you such a kind and caring person. Build an extra bedroom for your father and me, as we will be frequent visitors. Doris and Andy can sleep in the barn. Next week we'll be looking for a high speed buggy with four thoroughbreds."

The Johnsons found out how much they were loved by the town. Two days after the announcement of Nate is moving, there was a town party for him. There was dancing, good food, along with many laughs and smiles. Marjorie would have loved it; Nate did too. He even danced with his mother and sister. They also found out that six men and four wagons were ready to escort the Johnsons to Nate's new home. There was furniture, tools, hardware, and the blacksmithing items that Jack had given Nate years ago to be moved.

When Nate spoke to the large gathering, he mentioned that he was leaving some very special people in the best town on earth. He explained to them that his new town was calling him. He didn't know why, but he wanted to help Thomas make their new town as fantastic as this one is. Nate went on to say that, the people in this town are the best in the world, and then he repeated the words, the best in the world. This has been the greatest place to grow up, and it is all because of you. THANK YOU, THANK YOU, I LOVE YOU ALL. Mary just stood there crying remembering her eleven-year-old son at a town gathering holding hands with Marjorie as she spoke to him. OH MY

Nate drafted and sent a quick letter to Thomas the next morning after the party. It stated that the Johnson clan, four wagons, and six neighbors would arrive on the following Tuesday. He also said that the town gave him a party. It was a splendid time; he even danced and gave a little speech. He could not even count the number of people he hugged; there were so many. Marjorie would have been so proud.

Thomas wanted the arrival to be grand. The letter said that the caravan was leaving on Sunday after church. The vet figured the group would arrive around noon on Tuesday. He would have music and food ready when they arrived. He was excited to see everyone, especially Jeremy and M2. Thomas wanted the afternoon to be as festive as possible. It was going to be so much fun.

It was a grand reunion, with lots of laughs, smiles, and friendly conversation. The food was quite tasty. Everybody thoroughly enjoyed themselves. Thomas got the men rooms in town that came with a fine breakfast. He wanted these helpful men to enjoy a great night's sleep followed by a delightful start of the day at the best café in town. The Johnsons stayed in one of the spare bedrooms, and Nate, Doris, and Andy slept in the barn. This was Nate's idea. He said later that the three talked half the night away. It was so great visiting. All three laughed so much until Nate finally said that they needed to sleep.

The traveling party took off at 7:30 a.m. Thomas had been up since 5:30 fixing breakfast. It was served at 6:30, and the goodbyes started at seven. The vet thanked the Johnsons for helping with the move and making the whole trip so pleasant for the travelers. A couple of the men explained that Mary insisted on doing all the cooking with Doris and Andy's help. Jeremy led the men in campfire songs. It was very enjoyable. Thomas told the six men that he owed them, which they quickly dismissed. Each of them told the vet that they could never pay him back for all the things he had done for them; it was their pleasure to help. Jeremy shook the hand of his son's mentor and thanked him for giving Nate a place to start his next chapter.

The last person to approach Thomas was Mary. She pulled him aside and said, "I can't talk long but will write you a letter soon to say the things I need to. Yesterday when we arrived, I walked out to the side of the house. I still talk to Marjorie and probably always will. I think it is because there has never been anybody whom I enjoyed more than M. I made a comment to her that this would be a great spot for a garden. Thomas, she was there. Do you feel her here?"

"Yes I do, especially where you were standing," said the vet. "I haven't really wanted to start a garden, but today I do."

M2 added, "I believe someone from above wants you and Nate together again. Thank you, Thomas, for helping to give Nate a new beginning. I'll say more in my letter." She gave him a big hug and a peck on the cheek along with the words, "I love you."

Nate and Thomas started breaking ground for the garden that very day. Sharon, a distant neighbor, came by in her buggy. She stopped the buggy to say hello. Thomas waved and walked over to her. Nate followed. When the vet arrived next to Sharon's buggy, he smiled and said, "Good morning, Sharon. I want you to meet my assistant veterinarian, Nathaniel Johnson. He's moving into town and will be living with me for a while."

Nate walked over towards Sharon, stuck his hand out, and said, "Good morning, Sharon. It is nice to meet you. That is a fine buggy you have there and a good-looking mare. My friends call me Nate."

Sharon responded, "I will call you Nate then. Thank you for the compliment. They are my pride and joy. I see you men have quite a project underway. It is a great location for the garden. If I had the time, I would offer to help, but I am off to town to sell some jam. Well, good luck with your work and good day to both of you. It was nice to meet you, Nate."

After Nate finished his pleasantries with Sharon, he and Thomas started to leisurely go back to work. Thomas explained that Sharon and her husband live about a half mile away. He saw her one day on a buggy ride. He had taken a small road off the main one just to see where it went. He found two small ranches; Sharon was working in the garden at one of them. Thomas stopped and waved. Sharon came over and introduced herself. They have been friendly ever since. She is very pleasant to talk to. By the way, she makes the best jam in town.

Dan says that the husband was a very good rancher in the past but seems to have caught a couple of bugs. Nate jumped in to say how terrible that was, but the mentor went on to clarify these bugs were by the husband's own volition. He added the words, gambling and drinking. The husband has fallen behind in his work. The place looks in bad shape. The kind vet said that he even asked Sharon if he could help. She said that her husband wouldn't like that, but Sharon smiled and thanked him for the offer.

Dan says that the husband is usually pretty lucky at cards. In fact, he wins a fair amount from the storeowner and vet. Thomas said you couldn't always count on the cards for extra money. The tide sometime turns. The drinking is the real problem. The husband comes home very late and sleeps until nine; he does not start work until eleven. You know farmers and ranchers work a full day most often, especially in a two-person operation. Thomas felt so sorry for Sharon; she deserves better.

For the next several days, the two men worked on the garden, rode horses into the countryside, and made a lean to off the back of the barn for Nate's blacksmithing equipment. It was a very pleasant time, except when they traveled by Sharon's place. It was 10 a.m. Sharon was out working in the yard, and there was no husband in sight. Nate noticed that there was definitely lots of work that needed to be done. He felt so sorry for Sharon. She was doing the best that she could but needed help. He mentioned this to Thomas, and the mentor explained that not everybody has a good life. One of his goals is to make Sharon's a whole lot better. Nate simply said, "Agreed."

On Sunday Nate and Thomas attended church. Nate was hoping to get a look at Sharon's husband. That was rather difficult because neither Sharon nor her husband were in the church. After the service as the two vets were leaving, Nate said to Thomas, "Do you need a glass of water?"

Thomas laughed and explained, "I also do not care for this minister. I could talk about my dislikes for a long time, but maybe my saying that he was hired basically by "our" rancher friend will explain everything."

"I'm seriously considering not going back next Sunday," said Nate. "He was terrible."

No sooner than when the two got home and changed their clothes, Sharon came racing up to the house. She yelled that her husband's hurt. Please come. Thomas grabbed his bag from his buggy, as it was right next to him, jumped in Sharon's small two-seat buggy, and yelled for Nate to follow in Thomas' wagon. Nate was there five minutes after Thomas. He saw Thomas and Sharon facing towards him; the husband's body was behind them in front of the house. The vet was holding Sharon's hand. Both of them had their heads down; Nate knew what that meant. As Nate pulled up, Thomas sent Sharon into the house. She was gone for a few minutes, and when she came back outside the husband was already loaded in Thomas's wagon, covered by two horse blankets. Thomas had told Nate to take Sharon for a walk, keep her occupied with conversation, ride over to my place, and show her around. He would be back as soon as possible.

When Sharon approached Nate, he gave her a long hug and said how sorry he was. She had not cried yet. She might be in some kind of shock Nate thought. She held on for a longer time than Nate expected. He was not sure what to do. He did not really know her but started gently patting and rubbing her back.

Nate whispered the words, "I've got you."

Without letting up, Sharon said, "I'm all alone now."

Without knowing why, Nate held her tighter, gave her a kiss on the cheek, and replied, "You are not alone. You have Thomas and me. We are not going to leave you. You will have two best friends." He took her hand and continued, "Let's go for a short walk. When's the last time you walked with your best friend?"

"Never," she said.

Nate leaned over, kissed her other cheek and said, "That's from Thomas."

They walked in silence for a short distance as Nate caressed Sharon's hand. Then

Sharon started talking. She explained, "My husband shouldn't have been on the roof in his condition, but he could be very stubborn. Maybe I should have been more assertive, but sometimes he could get mean in his condition."

Nate stopped walking, took her back in his arms, and tried to comfort her. He said, "Sharon, This is not your fault in any way. My understanding is that some men are indeed stubborn and do not want to be told what to do. What your husband did was the result of who he was. In no way could you have stopped him. You might have even gotten hurt. Please realize this was out of your control."

Sharon kissed Nate on the cheek and said, "Thank you for those words. They make me feel better. You are a kind man."

Nate did exactly what Thomas had told him to do. He took Sharon back to Thomas' place after the short walk at her place. The kind young man showed her around and kept her busy with a flowing conversation. They held hands as they walked and talked. In the barn, Nate and Sharon fed and groomed the horse. They talked the entire time about what kind of work they enjoyed the most. Nate was very impressed that Sharon liked working with the cattle the most. The time flew by.

When Thomas returned three hours later, he told the others that he wanted to fix dinner. He said that he even had a nice bottle of wine. He said that he and Marjorie seldom drank wines in all their years together, but we all need one glass apiece. Nate, of course, had never had a sip of alcohol of any type, and Sharon had sipped some wine once or twice. They could not say no to such a charming man.

Thomas explained that since he has been in this town he has had wine about four times. Sleep seems to be much easier after a glass.

Thomas did indeed fix dinner. He would not take any help; he wanted Nate to keep Sharon busy with conversation. They did find several topics that interested of both them, horses and gardening. Dinner was served about an hour and a half later. Sharon and Nate couldn't believe that much time had passed. They had really enjoyed their conversation. Thomas poured the wine and the dinner was served. Thomas entertained with stories from his past vet practice experiences. He made the others smile, and it was a reasonably good time. Both men were very happy that Sharon was able to smile and enjoy dinner.

After dinner, Thomas shooed them into the living room. Sharon apologized for not helping with the dishes, but she needed to close her eyes for a few minutes. The vet took her to the spare bedroom. He said that he would wake her in ten minutes. He did not, and she slept until morning. Nate did the same in the other guest room. Thomas finished in the kitchen with a smile on his face. He felt sorry that Sharon had to go through this ordeal, but he wasn't unhappy at all about Sharon and Nate. He knew they would like each other. Fate had brought these two together. Thomas truly believed that these two were meant to be.

Chapter 10

Sharon

Sharon was going to stay at Thomas' place for a period. Thomas insisted, and Sharon didn't put up an argument. Each day the three went to Sharon's place to work, except for Tuesday. The first day Thomas and Nate looked at the place to see what lumber would be needed to fix up the ranch. The three spent some time ripping off the porch, as the wood, in Thomas' opinion, was rotten and dangerous. Sharon was concerned about the cost. She said that she wasn't even sure she would keep the ranch. The vet explained that if she did sell, she would get a better price if the place were in good working order. It's a nice ranch; it just needs some work.

He told Sharon that he was looking for a good project to occupy his time. He laughed and told her that he had told Nate that he would pay somebody to provide him with some good honest work. "You are doing me a huge favor." Thomas smiled and touched her shoulder as he finished his words.

Sharon's eyes watered some as she told them, "You are both too kind. You two have saved me from a very lonely and sad existence." She hugged them both as she gave them each a quick kiss on the cheek along with the words, "Thank you so much".

Thomas had talked to Dan after taking the husband to town. Dan knew everybody in town and offered to help with the arrangements. Thomas thanked him and then asked about the lumber situation in the neighboring town where the army was located. Dan explained that they have a great lumberyard with everything you will need. THOMAS WAS NOT GOING TO BUY ANY LUMBER FROM THE RANCHER. On Tuesday morning after an early breakfast fixed by Sharon, Thomas was on his way. He explained that he would be gone all day but hoped to be home by 6 p.m. Nate prepared the wagon while breakfast was being prepared. He had previously offered to make the trip, but Thomas insisted that he go.

Sharon's personable new "best friend" helped her clean up the kitchen after breakfast. Sharon smiled and commented that she had never had help doing the dishes before. Nate said that he was glad to help and mentioned that he could even cook some.

"Well, aren't you the handy one," said Sharon. "I think that is so wonderful. Who taught you, your mother? What other skills do you have, my new best friend, Nate?"

Nate smiled, "On my best days, I can crack an egg without it breaking into ten pieces. On my bad days, I usually drop it on the floor. I can also pour water into a bowl of flour without dropping the pitcher. I will tell you more as we work together today. I used to talk to my favorite mentor every day as we worked in the yard. I really enjoyed it. Talking while you work makes the work and the day much more pleasurable. I look forward to learning so much more about you as we talk our way through our work."

"I'm a pretty boring story," said Sharon. "I have spent most of my life doing chores around the house. I started from a very young age and have never stopped. I do have a surprise for you today. I also look forward to some conversation as, on most days, I work by myself. I will also put you in charge of pouring water," She smiled.

Nate liked the humor and the smile. He then pointed out, "Well, this is going to be a fun day with my new best friend, Sharon. By the way, I will always put my best foot forward when pouring water for you. I'll go get the buggy ready."

The two farm hands rode to Sharon's place with the conversation nonstop. Nate felt comfortable talking with Sharon. She did most of it because Nate was asking so many questions. He thought this would help her. He was pleased because Sharon was smiling some during the ride. This was a good sign. He hoped her grieving would be short-lived. Upon arriving at her place, Sharon excused herself for a moment. When she came out of the house, she had cowboy boots on, overalls, a light long sleeved blouse, and a cowboy hat. Nate started laughing and made the comment that she was the best-looking ranch hand he had ever seen. Sharon thanked him, touched her hat like the one cowboys do, and explained that this was so much more comfortable to work in and easier to clean. Her husband had not allowed it; he said it made her look like a man.

Nate quickly spoke, "Sharon, I have seen many cowboys on my vet visits, and none of them had as pretty of a face as you. No man has as pretty of a smile as you do; I might add. You are 100% gorgeous in whatever you wear. I'm excited to have such a good looking working partner."

"Thank you, Nate," said Sharon. "I haven't received such nice words," she paused, "in forever. Where do you want to start to work, my best friend?"

Nate took her hand, and they walked side by side to the barn where they cleaned stalls, fed animals, and straightened things out. They constantly talked about work. Nate made it clear that Sharon was in charge. He continued to ask many questions. The young man enjoyed getting to know his new friend. After they finished the barn work, they proceeded to the garden, house, and finished up with some fence repair. Sharon fixed a couple of sandwiches for lunch, and Nate made it a point to tell Sharon that he would pour the water.

She laughed and touched his arm. Nate liked that.

In the afternoon, the two ranch hands rode out to check the stock. They were going to move them to a different location. Sharon explained, "The cattle like a little box canyon where there's good grass and some protection from predators. That is where we are moving them. We have a fence to keep the herd in place. First, we'll move the herd into the coral where we can check them out." Nate and Sharon did, in fact, check the stock over together after getting them into the corral. Nate was impressed that his partner knew so much about cattle. They all appeared to be very healthy. Nate had not ridden horses much and wasn't nearly as quick and nimble as Sharon was on her horse. Nate did the best he could. He at least covered one side and made some noise. It was enough that Sharon was able to do most of the herding. He did get the corral gate opened. Sharon told him just before the move to the box canyon that the cattle like this canyon so much. When you open that gate, stand back because they will be rushing through to their favorite spots. She laughed when she said this. Nate liked it when she laughed.

When they got back, they groomed the horses while Nate mentioned to his good-looking partner that he needed to practice his herding skills. Sharon smiled and said that he did exceptionally well for his first attempt. He said that his goal was to be half as good as she was. Later, Nate chopped wood as Sharon visited with him. She wanted to help chop, but Nate said that he had a strong back and long arms for good advantage. He liked doing the work because it was a good workout, and the young repairperson said that he really liked Sharon visiting with him as he did it.

The afternoon went by quickly as both people seemed to be enjoying each other's company. They headed back around 3:00 to check Thomas' garden. A short time later, they both cleaned up and changed clothes. They met in the kitchen where Nate informed Sharon that he was going to fix one of Thomas' favorite dinners, and he would really like his new best friend to help.

Sharon asked Nate to please tell her how he came about learning to cook. Nate told her, "I had five great mentors in my life, Thomas, Jack, my mother and father, and the one who taught me the most amazing lessons of all, Thomas' wife, Marjorie. She is the one responsible for my cooking abilities, limited as they are. She told me that all men should know something about cooking, so I learned. She was a great cook and a wonderful teacher. I will tell you so much more about her as we spend more time together. She actually is the reason that you know Thomas and me." While Nate was talking, they were fixing dinner. There were a few laughs along the way, very pleasant for both of them. As dinner was simmering, Nate and Sharon sat on the porch discussing all the work they had done that day. Sharon mentioned that there has not been that much work done in a day at her place in a very long time. She thanked Nate as they were both walking in to check on dinner. They were both starving and could not wait for Thomas to arrive.

Sharon asked, "Is it okay to give my best friend a friendly thank you hug and a kiss on the cheek?" She smiled.

Nate replied, "That would be a great way to end a wonderful day. I loved working and talking with you today, Sharon."

The couple embraced, maybe for a little longer than they should have, but they both enjoyed it too much to cut it short. Sharon kissed Nate on his right cheek and Nate returned the favor twice. Nate was constantly caressing Sharon's back. She really liked that. Nate did too.

Dinner was very good. Thomas thanked Nate and Sharon several times. The conversation centered on Sharon's ranch. She explained what she and Nate had accomplished. Thomas was impressed. He said, "I know how good of a worker Nate is; you must be just as good. Isn't it great to do a good day's work? I can't wait for tomorrow. Nate's going to show me how to hit your thumb with a hammer." Sharon had a puzzled look on her face because Thomas and Nate were laughing. Nate explained the previous conversation with Thomas about his thumb and a hammer.

"Now I get the joke about the thumb and hammer. That would be a funny children's story about how a hammer and thumb become friends," said a smiling Sharon. "Nate, thank you for the wonderful dinner. I will do the dishes as you two talented men relax."

Thomas excused himself to go cleanup after thanking the two cooks. Once again, Nate joined his fellow cook in the kitchen where he helped her clean up. Both went to the porch to sit and talk some after completing their task. Thomas deliberately kept busy elsewhere. He had a sense of what was happening and was overjoyed that his "son" had met someone. As soon as the cooks sat down, Nate asked Sharon about her childhood. She explained that she was an only child; her dad had wanted a boy. He never paid much attention to her. He worked long hours as most farmers do. As soon as she was old enough, she joined him working the land and tending to the animals. She did her best to please her dad, but he never did appreciate all the work she did. She doesn't even remember any compliments at all. They didn't even talk much.

Nate reached over, took her hand, and said, "I mean no disrespect whatsoever, but you did everything right. Your father had a flaw. Let me ask you a question. I don't mean to pry, so if I am going too far with my questions, feel free to say so. Did your dad respect your mom and appreciate the work she did?"

"The answer is no, he did not," whispered Sharon. "I just thought with all my physical work he would appreciate me. You have given me more compliments in the last couple of days than I received from my dad the entire time growing up. It hurts me to think about it."

Nate explained, "Please don't think that you did anything wrong. I am going to tell you a shortened version of me when I was young. Between the ages of three and eleven, I did not talk much. I didn't like to touch people as in a hug or in some sign of affection. I didn't like to be touched. Therefore, I guess you could say I was flawed. When I was eleven, Marjorie Smith took my hands one day and told me that if I ever had any questions about things, I could ask her for help. At that moment something happened to me. I wanted her help. I knew that it would make me happier. For the next nine years, Thomas and Marjorie were my primary mentors. They were amazing and made me into the man I am today. My point is that your dad did not receive the mentoring needed to be able to appreciate others and give compliments. It was his flaw, not yours. Sharon, you are so easy to compliment because you do great things and are a pretty amazing person."

Sharon did not say anything. She reached over, took Nate's hand with both of hers, leaned in, and gave him a quick peck on the cheek. She put her head on his upper chest for a moment and then quietly said, "I don't feel alone anymore."

As Sharon sat up, Thomas walked out onto the porch. He announced that he was tired, so he was going to go to bed. He thanked them both again for dinner. He also mentioned that he was really looking forward to tomorrow. He did not tell them that the window was open, and he had heard their entire conversation. He didn't want to interrupt and couldn't leave because he wanted to hear everything. He went to bed a happy man.

On Wednesday, breakfast was quick and easy. The three loaded up the wagon with some more tools, hopped in the wagon, and were off to Sharon's place. The vet was excited to get started. He really missed working. Nate and Thomas spent most of the time repairing or replacing spots that were in disrepair. Nate was on the roof for quite a while. He really did a masterful job. His work with Jake had really paid off. Thomas had done a few porches in his lifetime, so he jumped right into cutting the pieces. The wood was dry and straight, top-notch building material. He still added two more cross members to help keep the wood from warping. He and Nate had agreed on that Monday.

Sharon worked in the garden and went to town per Nate's request to buy the ingredients for Thomas' favorite lunch. He didn't know the prices but gave her plenty of money. He completely trusted her. He felt that he and Sharon might be more than friends might. There was definitely a connection. Lunch was a total surprise for Thomas. He thanked Nate for being so thoughtful and Sharon for the preparation. The three smiled and laughed their way through lunch. Sharon wondered if these two friends always laughed so much. She was not used to it, but she definitely enjoyed it. It made the day and the work so much more pleasant. The men sure were good with hammers and saws. Everything was starting to look quite a bit nicer.

Thursday was another day of work at Sharon's place. Today was fence day. Nate started out by himself, as Thomas wanted to help Sharon check on the stock. When he got back from the ride, the men repaired so many fence posts they lost count. Sharon worked with the horses. They had leftovers for lunch. Thomas thanked her for giving him something to do. He enjoyed the work and loved the company. The three definitely got along well. Sharon really liked to be near people who laughed, smiled, and talked while they worked.

On Friday morning, Thomas had a meeting with Dan about their plan for replacing the town council. The personable vet was gone when the local minister pulled up to Thomas' place. He was dressed as he was ready to give the Sunday sermon. Nate thought that was strange. His father always dressed in regular clothes during the week. These clothes were much easier to work in, along with the idea of dressing up just on Sundays made that day quite special. His father liked that, so did his mom. Sharon was getting ready for the day. The minister was direct in his comments, assertive. He told Nate that having a single widow woman here in the house with a young single man was ungodly. It was a sin, and he would never allow anyone like that in his church. He finished with the words that Nate was not welcomed in his church. Nate quickly responded that Thomas and he were just trying to help a neighbor in need, but the minister was already walking off. Sharon was by the front door and heard everything.

On the ride to her place, Sharon mentioned what she heard. She said that she did not want to cause any trouble.

Nate responded, "We don't like him anyway; I wasn't going to go back this week." He also explained that maybe he wasn't completely honest with the minister. "It may be wrong to say, and I'm sorry if it offends you, but I like you, I think, more than a friend."

Sharon smiled and told Nate that she liked him too. She added, "I don't know what to do. Maybe Thomas might have some advice. My life has changed completely in just five days. It has been so fast that I'm overwhelmed."

Thomas rolled up in his buggy shortly after Nate and Sharon arrived in the wagon. They had just started with the animals. The young vet explained to his mentor what the minister had said. Thomas responded that he would take care of it at church on Sunday morning. He happily walked off to start on his work. The young couple did not say anything to the kind vet about their feelings for one another. Nate told Sharon that one problem at a time was enough? He quickly added, "My feelings for you are not a problem at all. They are my biggest joy. I have never been so happy in my entire life, but Thomas wants to handle the minister situation first. We'll ask for advice later."

Sharon told Nate that she had a situation that might be a problem. "Nobody knows about it, but you need to know. My husband's name was Bookings; my name is Sharon Ginger Taylor. We were never legally married. I'm so sorry if this is a problem for you."

Thomas had gone to a distant fence line over behind the house that kept the cattle in their rightful location. He was going to repair anything that needed addressing. He was so happy to have this work. He was also thrilled to have Nate and Sharon. He loved that the couple seemed to enjoy each other's company. His days were now a blessing.

Nate and Sharon were in the barn when Nate spoke, "Sharon Ginger Taylor, it is absolutely no problem for me. I am very fortunate to have met someone who is so very special in a number of ways. I've only known you for five days, but I could fill a page of paper describing how fantastic you are. I would have to write in very small print to get it all on one page," He smiled. Nate continued, "This has been a whirlwind for me too. I have never kissed a woman or girl before, except for family. I have never kissed a person on the lips. I'm a little nervous about it."

Sharon took his hands in hers and explained that he would soon experience that pleasure many times. They were in the barn and Thomas was still way out on the fence line... Sharon put both her hands on the sides of Nate's face, leaned forward, and gave her person his first real romantic kiss.

"That was utterly amazing, my dear Sharon," Nate said as he put his arms around her. "My heart is still racing. Maybe we can practice some more soon. Marjorie used to say that the more you practice the better you get. I want to be as good as you are. You were wonderful."

Sharon smiled, kissed Nate's cheek, and said, "You were wonderful."

Thomas went to town on Saturday to talk with Dan. He wanted the lawyer to introduce him on the porch of the church a few minutes before the doors opened. The minister did not like talking in his church, so he didn't let the people in too early. There was always a crowd of people waiting to get in. The lawyer agreed that the timing would be perfect. Thomas explained what he was going to say. The lawyer thought his friend's words were perfect. In addition, the people of the town would get a chance to meet the personable vet.

Thomas was outstanding in his speech. The lawyer thought he would never want to go against the vet in court. The people in attendance listened attentively and seemed to be in complete agreement with Thomas and Nate's actions. Toward the end of Thomas' speech, a man in the back spoke up. He explained that his friend knows Dr. Smith. The friend who lives in the doctor's prior town stated that the doctor and his late wife were the finest people that you could ever meet. They have created an atmosphere of love and kindness, along with the idea that helping a neighbor in need is, perhaps, one of the finest things a person could do. The whole town is a better place because of them. So many people have adopted their values. They have left a lasting legacy in that town that people talk about every day. The stranger in the back of the audience also stated that this town is lucky to have Dr. Smith and Nate Johnson here. Nate Johnson is an outstanding young man. Thomas thanked the man for his kind words.

The kind doctor had said no harsh words towards the minister. He quoted scripture, explained the situation briefly, and smiled before telling the audience that it felt so wonderful to help Sharon. She seems like a very nice woman. He apologized for interrupting their quiet Sunday morning but felt something had to be said. He thanked them for listening and said that he was going to host a Bible study with Nate and Sharon. It should be fun. Have a blessed day, everyone. With those words, Thomas mounted his buggy and drove home.

The crowd outside the church couldn't stop talking about the minister and Thomas. Dan chuckled several times to himself as he heard the discussions. It was all positive for the vet and overwhelmingly against the minister. Two couples left to go home. Dan knew right then the name of one of the new members of the town council, Dr. Thomas Smith. GOOD CHOICE.

When Thomas arrived back at his place, Nate and Sharon were dressed up some. The kind doctor had told his young protégé that he wanted to host a Bible study, just the three of them. Sharon had never been to church in her entire life. Thomas knew this already; he and Sharon had discussed church on a couple of occasions. She explained to both men that she was somewhat embarrassed about not knowing anything. The ever-kind vet stated emphatically that there is absolutely no reason to be embarrassed. You were never given the chance to learn, but now you have. It will be fun.

As Nate and Sharon started to sit at the dining room table, Thomas brought out

Marjorie is Bible and told Sharon that he would love her to have it because Bibles should be read and used often. Marjorie would have loved you, Sharon; she would want you to have this. Thomas picked out his favorite part of the "Good Book" to start the reading and discussion. The study went very well. Sharon was interested, did some reading, and asked several very good questions. All three agreed to do a study every Sunday morning.

Thomas shooed the young ones outside because he was fixing lunch. He was excited and felt quite warm. He knew who was there. The young couple held hands as they walked towards the garden. Sharon advised Nate that they needed to be careful about their affection for each other. He quickly agreed and stopped holding her hand. He said that this was going to be very difficult, but he understood completely. Sharon asked about Marjorie.

Nate explained, "Thomas and I think Marjorie was an angel sent down to earth to help people, and me in particular. To watch her with people was amazing. She had a smile that would warm up a room. Marjorie always spoke kind and loving words. My mother also thinks it is possible that she was an angel. My mother was an only child. One day as they were hugging goodbye, my mother whispered that she loved Marjorie, but she used M instead of her name. From that day forward, my mother loved M as a big sister. My mother's name is Mary, so M called her M2. They really loved each other. It was so touching to see them talk to each other."

"It's hard to believe, but I feel her here in the garden. She really liked gardening. We worked hundreds of hours together in her and Thomas' garden. Thomas believes that Marjorie's work on earth is not complete. She will not leave until it's done. I will share many of her lessons with you because she taught me things that prepared me for you, my love."

Sharon simply said to Nate, "Follow me."

When they got inside the barn, Sharon kissed Nate. Then she asked him to teach her one lesson right now if he wanted. Nate said that couples sometimes have special language between them, some unspoken, and some spoken. No one else knows this special communication. It is just between the couple. Having this unique language makes their relationship very special, intimate. It strengthens their bond and allows the couple to reach the highest level of love. It is the greatest feeling a person can ever have. Our Lord has given that to us to have as a couple. Your last name is Taylor. When we are alone, when we are holding each other, or when we are talking in private while we work, I will whisper "T" to you. It is meant to say to you that "I love you, I adore being near you, I love being part of us, and I will always feel our connection." With those words, Nate hugged Sharon and whispered, "T, I love hugging you." He didn't let go for quite a while. Sharon did not say anything. She just gave her person a long romantic kiss.

When the three met up for lunch, Thomas explained to Nate and Sharon, "I am the new owner of five acres of land. The army will be rolling in on Wednesday to start construction on several buildings: a reception area and office, barracks, kitchen with attached mess hall, and a rather large barn. They will also have to figure out how to incorporate a plan to make it all look good. Dan gave me some plans for the buildings on Friday. I would like Nate to look them over during lunch. We could use his design skills and construction know-how."

"The Colonel who's leading the construction group was an engineering major at West Point. He knows what he is doing, but I thought we should have a basic idea of what is needed and where to put things. They are bringing two large wagons full of wood and tools. Once these items are unloaded, the wagons will make several more trips to bring in all the items needed for the outpost. I thought we could ride out today to view the property and discuss where to put the buildings." Sharon told Thomas that the trip sounded like fun; she would love to go.

Nate added, "Well, I'm home, and I have some work to do. I guess you could say its homework. It's due in thirty minutes, so I had better get started. I hope I get a good grade." He smiled.

Thomas and Sharon talked about the troops coming to town. He also mentioned that Dan and he, along with three other men, were running for town council. Sharon thought that was a splendid idea. Some people don't really care for the existing town council. You should be the town's representative. You are very well spoken and have a gift with people. It would be so great for this town if you were in charge.

Thomas held her hand and said, "My Marjorie was the town spokesperson. She taught everyone so much about love, kindness, and doing good deeds. I have always been a good person; Marjorie made me better. We used to talk about Nate every evening when we were his official mentors. She guided me. You have met one amazing young man, so kind and loving. He has a great work ethic, is highly skilled, and is of the highest moral character."

Sharon whispered, "He's also very handsome with a great physique."

Thomas laughed and said, "Oh, you noticed?" The vet smiled. "He's very easy to like."

Sharon glanced over at Nate who was busy writing on the side of the paper that contained the building plans. She turned back to her kind host and explained that she might have noticed that Nate was easy to like. She smiled and touched Thomas' hand. He quickly thought that she has some of the same mannerisms as M. How lucky for Nate.

The three "building developers" headed over to the property. They started walking around when Nate asked about the property lines. The senior member of the group explained, "The rancher was very happy with the sale. He said that the land does not grow anything, and it is worthless to him. He actually thought it might be a good place for a couple of buildings. He stated that he was not concerned about a few feet here or there. Your question is a very sound one, spoken like a lawyer. We will mark three of the boundaries with rocks today, the fourth being where the two roads cross. Good thinking, Nate." The three continued to look around discussing where to place the buildings. Nate made the comment that you should always build more than you think you need. In the end, you always could use more. Jake taught me that.

As the three visitors finished placing the rocks, Thomas explained that he would draw up a document that he and the rancher would sign before Wednesday. Nate had walked off the distances and marked everything down. Everybody really enjoyed their time looking around and talking. Sharon especially thought it was great because she had been treated as an equal. The men asked her opinions about things and listened to what she said. This had never happened before. NEVER!

Chapter 11

Big Events

Soon after the construction started on the new military outpost on the land furnished by Thomas, the questionable rancher showed up to talk with the man in charge. The rancher welcomed the Colonel to town, introduced himself, and explained who he was. He offered his assistance if any was needed. He also mentioned that he was the local blacksmith and lumberman. The rancher did not like the idea that the military was so close by. He ran the show around these parts. Now he would have to deal with Colonel Jones and his men. He couldn't do much because the town limits were drawn up a couple of years ago. This property was just outside the limits. He sensed that this was deliberate. He was a smart man and knew that the new vet and his friend Dan were behind the building of this outpost. He also knew that both men were running for town council. The election was about two months away, and the rancher would have to get to work leveraging votes. He knew it might get ugly. That's why he didn't want the military so close.

Nate decided to build two fire pits, one for Thomas and a bigger one for the outpost. They were both capable of cooking food. During the last two months while living on what is now Jack and Mabel's property, he built one for his mother. She loved it and would use it during the summer when it was so hot in the house. The family had always enjoyed an occasional fire in the evening. M2 mentioned that it would be very nice to sit in close proximity to the fire while everybody enjoyed visiting.

Nate thought it would be nice if he built a portable fire pit for the military outpost. The soldiers would get the benefits of cooking outdoors and enjoying a fire after a tough day of work around the area. The town market could also use it. Being portable allowed it to be moved into the barn or outside, depending on the weather. The barn was vented in the loft with four windows and had four doors on the bottom level. Colonel Jones and Nate had agreed to build an extra-large barn. The officer knew that it would be where the town market would take place. He liked the idea of people gathering in and around the barn. The men were often bored with nothing to do during their off duty time. They would surely enjoy the activity.

Thomas and Dan liked the aspect of the market being outside of town where all the farms and ranches were. It made it easier for them to bring their goods to the market. Town people could walk or buggy out to the market. The military's presence would provide extra safety in and around town. Dan had previously told the Colonel all about the rancher who ran the town to benefit himself and his "cronies". This is why there were always two guards on duty every night. The Colonel was not going to let a bully and crook attack his command and the good things that Dan and Thomas were trying to accomplish in this developing town. He knew Dan quite well and admired the kind of person he was. Thomas also impressed him.

Dan told Nate that he owned some land out a ways from town. It was fenced and locked with no trespassing signs. It had some old mining equipment lying around and a number of old buildings. The lawyer said that Nate could take anything he could use. Dan really liked the idea of a portable fire pit and knew the Colonel would agree.

Nate and Sharon went out a few days later to salvage whatever they could. They found some great pieces of iron, enough to make both fire pits. What Nate really enjoyed was the alone time with Sharon. They talked, laughed, held hands, and had several romantic moments where Nate whispered T several times at just the right moment. Sharon loved her new nickname. She could tell that when Nate called her T, it was full of affection. After one particular embrace, Sharon whispered, "Can I call you J?"

His response spoke volumes. Tenderly stroking her face with one hand, a kiss on the cheek, forehead to forehead, both hands caressing her, a kiss on the lips, followed by the words, "T, I would love that." Neither person had ever been so happy.

Thomas and Sharon took on all the chores when Nate started blacksmithing. Jack had given Nate some pointers when the skilled apprentice built his mother's fire pit. He remembered everything and knew he could produce a quality product. Not only did he want to impress the Colonel, he wanted Thomas to see the work he could do by himself. He was extremely motivated.

Sharon dropped by every day after her chores were done to see how things were going. Some days it would be at the post where Nate and Thomas were working or at Thomas' place in the blacksmithing area. Nate loved her coming by. It was always the highlight of his day. After a couple of days of not being alone at all with Sharon, Nate explained to Sharon that sometimes he really needed to clean up after blacksmithing because it is such physical work. Sharon laughed and stated that she was aware of the condition. Nate quickly apologized.

T smiled and said to her person, "There's no need to apologize. I love you every minute of every day, no matter how hard you have worked."

"Well, in that case, can you follow me to the barn for a minute?" Said Nate. The blacksmith hadn't hugged Sharon in two days. He had really missed it.

She followed a ways behind just in case someone was walking or riding by. The couple had done so well hiding their relationship. There was no reason to mess it up now. When they got inside, Nate said that he had a pain in his chest. He stated that he didn't know what it was, but maybe a quick hug would help. Sharon obliged. Nate said that the pain was gone.

"You are going to be my new doctor," Nate said as he smiled. "You do wonders for my heart. Seriously, I miss working with you and look forward to your dropping by every day. I just wanted you to know that. I love your company."

Sharon replied that she missed Nate just as much. Thomas is wonderful in so many ways, but he is not my Nate.

Nate took her hands, kissed the back of them, and said, "T, thank you for those words. Years ago, I heard Marjorie say 'my Thomas' to me as we were visiting. I really liked those words, 'my Thomas'; it explained so much about them. I always wondered if I would ever have that type of relationship, and today you said 'my Nate'. Those words make me love you more today than yesterday, and I don't know how that's possible." The young couple kissed and left the barn ten feet apart. A short time later, Nate started to think about how special his conversations with Sharon were. He couldn't believe how naturally he used M's lessons. Nate had explained a few to Sharon. She seemed to really like Marjorie's lessons.

The next day while doing chores, Thomas asked Sharon just how much she loves Nate. He laughed at the look on her face and explained that he'd known for some time. He also stated that he was so happy for both of them. He went on to say that, Dan says there is no legal time to wait, but it is customary not to remarry for a year. He did explain that in your case he thinks six months would be adequate.

The kind vet explained that after meeting you and visiting on numerous occasions, he knew that Nate would really like you. Thomas said that he has known Nate for virtually his entire life. M taught him about the love of a spouse and how special it is. Nate will explain many things to you as taught to him by Marjorie. He has been waiting for the right person to come along. Sharon, you are that person. When your life paths crossed, they aligned, and your destinies blended into one. He has never been so happy. You are going to love his family. They are going to love you. It will be a blessing for everybody. You and Nate will be very special together.

He explained, "I was drawn to this town and believe it was my job to bring you two together. Maybe Nate has told you that we believe that my wife was an angel put on earth to do great things. She absolutely did. She did so much for so many, and the last thing she did was to put you two together through me. I don't profess to know what two is in store for you, but I feel the love you two have for each other will radiate outwards and affect many others."

Sharon simply said, "I have never been so happy. Every day I love Nate a little more. Is that possible?"

Thomas replied, "Yes it is, Sharon. I am not an authority on the subject, but from my personal experience, it is entirely possible. M and I shared a love that was so intertwined with each other. I loved her good deeds and the help she provided for others. She loved what I did. There was never any jealousy or hard feelings about what we did independently. Together we did great things. Marjorie did things for me; I did things for her. Every night when we got into bed, we both felt that we were blessed to have had such a great day doing good deeds and being a positive influence. This is what I see for you and Nate."

Sharon didn't talk. She just hugged Thomas. She wanted to ask just how hard is it to go on without Marjorie but thought that would be inappropriate. Thomas knew what was likely going through Sharon's mind and spoke to that subject. "Sharon, it's been four months since my wife went back to heaven. The first month was difficult. I struggled but was lucky to have family nearby. Nate was especially helpful as was his mother. Nate told me to talk to Marjorie. He explained that he has learned to really enjoy it. It brings back memories of lessons, smiles, hugs, and laughter. I have come to experience the same enjoyment. I would not change one thing in my life. I was truly blessed to have M for thirty-three years. I am also blessed to have you and Nate here. Plus, you gave me something to do, and I needed that. Sharon, the best thing by far, you are completing Marjorie's and my 'son'. Every night as I get into bed, I think of my good deeds for the day along with being a positive influence. I also think of you and Nate," said an emotional Thomas.

"Marjorie sounds like she was truly amazing. I only hope I won't be a big disappointment," said a teary-eyed Sharon.

Thomas took her hands and quietly said, "You don't have to be Marjorie. Be yourself. You are a perfect fit for Nate. You will learn from each other, work together, and, most importantly, you will love each other more than anything else will in this world. I know Nate cherishes you so much, and I think you cherish him. This is so special. Again, you are meant to be together."

"Thank you for such kind words, Thomas," responded a touched Sharon. "I have been so lucky to have met two such wonderful gentlemen."

"Soon you'll meet some more," said a smiling vet.

The two workers went back to chores. They both were quiet for a few minutes as they were reflecting on the just finished conversation. Both were thrilled with what was said. On the way back to Thomas' place, Sharon told her work mate that she really enjoyed his company today and all the kind words. Thomas didn't answer; he just reached over, held her hand for a while, and squeezed it several times. As soon as the workers arrived "home", Sharon jumped out of the buggy and headed straight for Nate. Thomas only smiled as he watched her pull Nate into the barn. They didn't come out for a few minutes.

The fire pits were done and Nate was very proud of his work. The workmanship was superb. He couldn't wait for everyone to see them. As he was making them, he realized that he actually wanted Sharon's approval more than Thomas' or the Colonel's. Sharon couldn't stop smiling and saying great things about the fire pits.

Thomas was more reserved probably because he did not want to interrupt Sharon's reaction. He envisioned this happening hundreds of times where one gets so excited about the other's work. These two young people had such great things to give. After things settled down, Thomas calmly said, "Nate, you are a true craftsman. Whenever you see a work of yours, you definitely should be proud. It is such a beautiful piece." He then said to

Nate, "Go get cleaned up because Sharon and I are fixing dinner."

It took three weeks for the outpost to be completed. Before construction began, Nate had suggested putting the mess hall right behind the combination colonel's office and reception office. The Colonel loved the idea. The men built a nice indoor walkway connecting the two buildings. The front of the office was very nice. Nate and Thomas, who both helped build it along with some of the more skilled soldiers, had designed it. Colonel Jones was very impressed with everything. These two men had done so much fantastic work. He walked over to Nate and Thomas to thank them for such an amazing job. As they started shaking hands, Thomas asked the Colonel to please follow. He explained that Nate has built your post something.

When the Colonel saw the fire pit, he was very impressed. He couldn't stop talking about the workmanship. The men will really enjoy this. He thanked both men for everything they had done; from the buying of the land and building materials; to the building of the fire pit, and everything in between. It took him several minutes. The Colonel mentioned that Dan had said that he knew two men who would be able to help in the building and design of the outpost, but the senior soldier had no idea just how talented these two would be. Men, you have amazing talents; your design skills and carpentry expertise are professional quality.

Nate pointed out that we have a good source of wood, but we do need a large heavy wagon along with an adequate supply of muscle. Colonel Jones replied, "Men, I will be leaving in the morning, back to my old duty station. This billet is suited for a lieutenant. I have a good one coming in today. I will fill him in on everything. He will accommodate your request for men and a wagon. I will also explain that he is to be helpful in regards to all future market days and the planning that goes into them. I plan to be here for the first one. When is it?"

Thomas replied, "Two weeks from Saturday."

"See you then and good luck with everything," said the Colonel as he shook hands again with Nate and Thomas.

Plans were made later that day for a detail of men, plus Thomas, Nate, and Sharon to harvest wood at Dan's property on Friday. Thomas had already talked to the Colonel about soldiers doing some local work when they were off duty. The Colonel really liked the idea, especially at this outpost, as there was not much to do as far as assignments were concerned. The rancher who sold the acres to Thomas for the outpost told the Colonel that army horses could graze on the land nearest the outpost. He didn't use it anymore as it was too far away. There were only ten horses at the outpost. The Colonel authorized the purchase of several more horses depending on what the Lieutenant saw fit. Most days were slow for the majority of the troops. Every day there was work for three cooks and four men to handle the horses. Patrols hadn't started as of yet. The soldiers welcomed something to do.

The Colonel set up a plan where the soldiers could work with the public. If the troops were on duty, they would keep half of the pay with the other part going to enhance their rations. The Colonel knew the army didn't provide enough money to give the men something special now and then. If the soldiers were off duty, they kept all the money. The officer emphasized that all men were to be on their best behavior when dealing with the public.

Thomas arranged for two men to stay at Sharon's place and two at his own place for Friday's excursion to Dan's property. He wasn't taking any chances with the rancher. The vet knew the feelings between him and the rancher were mutual. Dan knew so many people in town who disliked the "town bullies". They kept Dan apprised of the rancher's movements, along with the sheriff's discussions with any newcomers to town. The lawyer, in turn, kept Thomas informed of the situation. Dan had even brought in a hired gun to act as a personal assistant. Nobody knew. Dan explained to his vet friend that he believed that Thomas didn't need to hire anyone. To this date, Dan wasn't aware of any activity by the sheriff or the rancher. They just might be a little too confident in their bid for reelection.

The men Thomas hired would tend to the horses, work in the garden, and chop some wood. It was not to be a day full of work. They were mostly there to guard the place.

Weapons were a necessity, but Thomas didn't expect any difficulties with soldiers nearby.

The Lieutenant had been briefed on the situation with the bully rancher. Sharon's place was fairly close to the outpost; the men could actually walk to the job. Thomas told the men they might want to ride to his place. The vet would pay the men well as was his style.

Friday was going to be fun. Thomas figured that if everyone chipped in with the work, it would be done just before lunch. Dan was also coming with his super sharp two-man saw and a helper named Ed. The army was bringing two saws. There would be six people cutting, and Dan, Ed, and Sharon handling the stacking. After lunch, Thomas wanted to teach Nate and Sharon how to shoot a rifle. Lunch was just fruit and jerky, but Thomas said he would buy everyone a nice dinner in town after a shooting contest. It was all going to be so much fun.

Thomas brought five top-notch rifles and two fine pistols for the friendly competition. Nate had seen the gun cabinet in the Smiths' bedroom but never thought much of it. He figured that Thomas' dad must have shot. Boy was he wrong. Everybody was invited to shoot. The soldiers were okay with the rifles. Nate and Dan were beginners, and it showed. Dan's friend didn't want to shoot for some reason. Nobody asked as it wasn't their business. Not everybody likes to shoot. Nate said no at first but was convinced by Thomas to learn. It is good that a man knows how to shoot some. He didn't know, at that moment, just how well Sharon shot. Sharon and Thomas were experts. Who would have known? Thomas explained that his dad's hobby was shooting rifles and pistols. He won many awards.

Thomas continued, "He taught me to shoot, and I competed until Marjorie and I were married. I have never shot since but always told Marjorie that, if need be, I would shoot anyone to protect her. I always took a rifle and a pistol on our Sunday buggy rides. I have always believed that a man has to protect his family, but I stand corrected. Sharon, you are a wonderful shot. Who taught you to shoot?"

Sharon, in her cowgirl outfit, looked adorable. She answered, "My dad taught me. He needed two rifles shooting in case of emergencies. He told me, 'Your mother can't shoot at all, so you're nominated.' "I, like Thomas, used to compete. I did well in most competitions I entered. And like my dear friend, I quit after getting married."

"Can you quick draw?" asked Thomas.

"I can," said a smiling Sharon.

Thomas set up the competition. He thought twenty paces would be a good distance. Everybody has to practice their drawing with an unloaded pistol. The competition involved drawing your weapon and being the first to hit the target. There were eight shooters. Two soldiers, Thomas, and Sharon made it pass the first round. In the next round, both soldiers missed the target, so it was Thomas against Sharon in the finals. Thomas said that he needed an age handicap. He wanted Sharon to draw with her left hand. Everybody laughed. Thomas knew he was in trouble; Sharon was fast. She did in fact win. Thomas was a good sport. He said that he was happy for Sharon, but she had better be ready for a rematch. He explained that he was going to practice twenty-five hours a day.

Everybody packed up after a relatively fun day. The shooting was great. Nate said that he wanted to get much better. Everybody said that Sharon was fantastic. She thanked everybody but seemed somewhat embarrassed about it. Both Thomas and Nate sensed it. On the way home, Nate asked her about it. Sharon explained that her dad called her a freak of nature after many shooting events. It always hurt her feelings. She guessed she still gets a little embarrassed about the whole thing, but she still likes to shoot.

Nate quickly took her hand and said, "I am so sorry that happened. He was jealous of you. What he said was completely wrong for so many reasons. I love all your talents. You have taught me a number of things already. I am thrilled that we get to share what we know. I am looking forward to you teaching me how to shoot. You are an amazing woman; beautiful on the outside and wonderful on the inside."

Sharon leaded over and kissed Nate on the lips. Nate was surprised, but the champion shooter explained that Thomas knows about us. The vet smiled and nodded his head. He didn't want to interrupt. Nate went on to explain that he had learned so much from Marjorie and his mother. Women are to be valued and are the equal to men. Thomas taught me that. He further explained that he didn't mean physically, but all around. Women have the knowledge and the skills to be treated as equals. My father learned from Thomas to treat my mother more of an equal than he did in the past.

Dinner was very pleasant. The group had to be split up as the restaurant didn't have their table of nine available, but it had two tables that would work. The soldiers enjoyed being on their own. Thomas was sure they were using soldier language as they talked about the events of the day. They kept their voices down, but the vet noticed there was a lot of laughing. They deserved a good time as they had all done good work today.

Dan mentioned that Nate and Sharon were welcome to help themselves to more iron if they needed it. He said that they were actually at the small part of the mine on the first salvaging trip. Around the mountain, there are twice as many buildings. The rest of the conversation at the table centered on the election coming up in about five weeks. Thomas already knew that the town folks did not care for the current town council, but Dan explained this and a couple of other things to Nate and Sharon. Ed was working with some people to gather votes. Everyone in town knew not to public ally go against the council. There was much quiet talk about the election; Ed had many votes lined up. Dan also mentioned that Ed was an excellent shot and fast with a gun. Ed quietly said that he was no match for the pretty woman in the cowboy hat. Everybody smiled.

Upon arriving back at Thomas' place, the vet thanked the young couple for their help. He also thanked Sharon for the shooting lesson.

He was smiling when he said that. He added that he was glad she won. He touched her shoulder and told her that she was a joy to have on the excursion today. After he went inside, Nate and Sharon sat on the porch as it was still early evening. They both had something they wanted to talk about.

Sharon stated, "Nate, when you were talking about women and men being equals, my heart was bursting with love for you. That was such a fantastic thing. I wanted to tell you how much I loved you, but I didn't know if it was okay with you with Thomas present. I was thinking that in these situations I would squeeze your hand three times. The squeezes mean 'I love you'."

Nate quickly squeezed Sharon's hand three times. Then he said, "I'm so lucky to have you. When you won the shooting contest, I wanted to say how much I loved you. I had the same feelings as you, but now I will squeeze your hand in public. I hope they don't get too sore from me always squeezing them." He smiled, leaded over, and kissed her. Nate started caressing the back of Sharon's hands, his eyes watered up, and he whispered, "After the first town market, I want to take you to meet my family. Is that okay?"

Sharon gave Nate a long kiss and then said, "That's a big step."

Nate took a deep breath. He gathered himself and said, "The first of many – The only thing I care about is taking all of my steps for the rest of my life with you by my side." The couple hugged for the longest time with multiple kisses and caresses. There didn't need to be any words. Words would get in the way of the strong feelings between the two. They would, in fact, walk side by side, hand in hand, for the rest of their lives.

The town market was the big event on Saturday. The Colonel came in on Friday with five pounds of coffee and a giant pot. The farmers and ranchers were ready to bring their wares to market. The army cooks had everything ready for their stew. Nate and Sharon were ready with their biscuit ingredients and jam. The market opened at eight. The signs in town said, "Bring your mug and we'll fill 'er with free coffee – one free biscuit and jam to every attendee."

There was a large crowd, and everybody seemed to have smiles on their faces quite often. The Colonel seemed to think there was more talking and visiting than sales. The Colonel was concerned, but Thomas explained it wasn't about the sales as much as it's about the town enjoying each other's company. Good things will result from this gathering; Thomas guaranteed. The officer did notice that there were many biscuits, cups of coffee, and bowls of the army's stew being served. The army charged for their stew. The Lieutenant felt this was the right thing to do. Both officers felt the food and drink were contributing to the many smiles and friendly conversation.

Thomas and the Colonel did take note of the four "amigos" strolling around. The rancher, hardware owner, minister, and sheriff kept to themselves. Not once were they involved in conversation outside their little group. They didn't appear happy, especially the hardware store owner. He knew the store next door to his general store where he sold homemade goods at quite a markup was in serious trouble. The four council members did not stay long. After a brief conversation among the four with the rancher doing most of the talking, they left. Thomas and Colonel Jones observed the entire conversation from afar.

Thomas was thrilled with everything and figured the next one just a week before the election would really help the chances of the challengers in the town election. People sure seemed to enjoy the young couple making the biscuits. Nate and Sharon smiled and were very friendly to everyone. The biscuits and jam were top quality. Everybody loved them.

On Sunday morning, Nate and Sharon took off for Nate's family. They apologized to Thomas for missing Bible study but wanted to get on the road. Thomas said that he completely understood. He also gave those two rifles and a pistol for the trip. The couple arrived at the Johnson home Tuesday morning.

After introductions, everybody sat down to a very nice breakfast prepared by Mary and the kids. Nate had written to his mother right after the conversation with Sharon about bringing her home to meet his parents, so the family knew a few things about Sharon. Mary made everybody very at ease with her marvelous skills of conversation. Mary had told the family not to mention any questions about Sharon's age or the fact that she had been married. This would be highly inappropriate, as Nate had mentioned not to discuss these two things. Mary did notice that her son's face lit up when he touched Sharon's arm or shoulder. She knew this was the ultimate completion of her son from M's lessons about the love of a spouse. Sharon seemed perfect.

Wednesday morning after a quick breakfast fixed by Sharon and Mary, Nate and his father went into town to run some errands. In reality, there were no errands. Jeremy had told his son last year that, if he wanted it, he could have his great grandmother's wedding ring for his bride, when he found one. In town on this very special day, he showed the ring to Nate. It was gorgeous. Nate absolutely loved it. The local banker had been keeping it in his safe all these years. Nate would ask Sharon this afternoon. Mary and the kids didn't know.

The Johnson men saw Jack and Mabel in town, and Nate asked them to please be gone from home between 1 p.m. to 2 p.m. Jeremy asked Nate about talking to Sharon's dad about marriage, but Nate explained that it wasn't necessary. Nate told his father that he wanted to propose in the garden where M had taught him so many lessons about love. She would be there; she would be so happy.

After a quick lunch, Nate and Sharon went for a walk. They held hands as Nate explained how many thousands of times he had walked this same path to the Smiths' house. Upon arriving, he took her to the garden where Sharon commented on how well done everything looked. Nate explained that Mabel was very good at gardening. He didn't elaborate much as he had something else on his mind. Nate took Sharon in his arms and gave her a kiss.

He said, "I feel Marjorie here today. I guess it's only fitting that she would be here." He knelt down on one knee and asked, "Sharon Ginger Taylor, would you make me the happiest man on earth by marrying me?" He presented her with the ring.

Sharon took the ring and Nate's hands. She was so excited that she started jumping up and down several times. As Nate stood up, Sharon grabbed him and said, "Yes, yes, yes!" The young couple was shedding tears of joy as they continued to hug and kiss. Jeremy and Mary were also crying as they had been watching the entire event from the trees behind Nate's previous cabin.

There was great joy at the Johnson home. On the walk back, Nate and Sharon decided not to wait six months to marry. After the election, they would travel back here. It would be only fitting that Jeremy marry these two in the church Nate grew up in. It was going to be a very small wedding. Only the most important people in Nate's life would attend. Mary would handle all the arrangements, nothing fancy. Nate also knew that M would be there; she wouldn't miss it.

Thomas was elated about the news. Nate told him that the wedding was thirty-two days away. The vet couldn't get over how happy the couple was. He loved the ring and, of course, asked if he could do anything. Nate mentioned that Thomas could bring that splendid smile of his.

Over dinner, Thomas caught the couple up on all the latest news. Ed was doing a great job in town; there were many votes lined up. The vet and storeowner were distancing themselves from the rancher and sheriff. He explained that a few people had thanked him for the town market. It was his understanding that the next one was going to be even bigger. He mentioned that this time he wanted to pay Nate and Sharon for their time in addition to what he had done last time. It would give him great pleasure to do this. The vet also mentioned that the army was going for more wood on Wednesday. Lieutenant Haynes wants to stockpile as much wood as possible in the corner of the barn. He thanks you for helping to make the barn extra-large. Thomas told Sharon that the two soldiers who stayed at her place for the entire week really liked what they saw. There was even some discussion about buying the place after their service time is up. The place looks great. They took great care of everything.

Sharon said, "Thomas, thank you so much. How can I ever repay you for all that you have done?"

The kind man reached over, took her hand, put it in the middle of the table, put Nate's hand on top of Sharon's and said, "You already have."

The chores were pretty much caught up. Both places were in tiptop shape. With some extra time on his hands, Nate decided to build a birdhouse at Sharon's place for the next town market while she did a few chores. Periodically, she dropped over to watch him work. Once again, she was amazed at how talented he was.

She commented, "I love watching you create such wonderful things."

"Thank you," said Nate. "Do you want it? I can make another."

"You don't have time. I have plans for you, maybe some other time," said a smiling Sharon. She took him into the barn for a short time.

The town market was excellent, bigger, better, with many more products for sale. People responded by purchasing almost everything including Nate's birdhouse. Thomas walked around visiting with many people. Lieutenant Haynes was extremely organized. Everything went off like clockwork. He had more soldiers involved, and they seemed to be really enjoying the local folks. The young officer kept an eye on the four amigos when they showed up. They did not stay long. The lieutenant was glad there were soldiers at Sharon and Thomas' places.

As Election Day neared, the rancher and his "cronies" were not happy, especially the rancher. His mood at home resulted in horse whippings, yelling at his wife, and pushing his boys to do more work than normal. On Friday morning, there were storm clouds quite a ways off in the distance. The lumber mill needed logs. The rancher decided if they left now, they could beat the storm. The mountain dirt road wasn't usable to haul wood after a storm for about a week. They had to go now. He did not want people to start going to the lumber mill that Thomas had used. He heard through his sources that some were thinking about using that lumberyard. There were three large new wagons in town that he didn't control. He also knew that some of the soldiers were working with the public. He didn't need the army going after wood for the civilians. He also saw the portable fire pit. His empire was starting to crumble. He would definitely fight back. He knew the ranchers backed him. He controlled them. The sheriff had agreed to help sway the town vote. He had already started bullying some.

The rancher and his two sons took off for the mountains nearby to harvest some good dry wood that the rancher had seen on their last trip. One son mentioned that the area was further away than normal, and with the rain on the way, maybe they should wait. The rancher just called him a few names and that was the end of the conversation.

The lumbermen were quite surprised when they got deep into the mountains because it had rained considerably last night. The conscientious son was concerned, but his dad said that they would be fine. It was going to be difficult getting the wagon into the area to initiate the work, but the rancher was determined. He was the type that when angry or in a bad mood, he became stubborn and aggressive. He definitely was angry with Dr. Thomas Smith.

This old part of the road hadn't been used much because it was quite rocky. You could easily damage a wagon, but the men pushed on. The trees were high quality, straight and solid. For some reason they appeared to be dying, probably due to a lack of water. This was a natural occurrence in the forest. Once a tree dies, the wood starts to deteriorate over a period. The rancher was glad they were harvesting the trees now, instead of later, because there might not be a later.

The men worked hard, but the wood was surprisingly dense. The workers could see the rain clouds overhead; this was definitely a bad sign. Both sons wanted to get off the mountain. They didn't want to be going down these roads with a load of heavy wood in the rain with their dad in a bad mood. The dad insisted that the work continue even when the rain started. The men worked harder and got all the cutting and loading done. They quickly put the cover on the wagon and headed down the mountain road. It had been raining hard for about thirty minutes. One son mentioned leaving the wagon behind and riding the horses down, but the dad said that was a stupid idea.

The going was slow because of the rocks. The sons were constantly using long poles as levers to help advance the wagon. The rancher was getting angrier and angrier. Finally, the group hit the better part of the road, but it was quite flooded. Now both sons wanted to stop, but their dad said to get in the back and shut up. In the rain, the wagon brakes were not as effective, especially with the very heavy load. With the road flooded completely in spots, the inevitable happened. The wagon and men went off the edge. They didn't have a chance.

The rancher's wife expected her men home at about 5 p.m... At 6:00, she was starting to worry. By 7:00, she figured they had hunkered down for the night. She knew her husband wanted to be back for the election, but things happen. She really didn't care about the election. She secretly didn't approve of her husband's methods. In fact, she didn't care for her husband. Their love had died years ago. She was still trying to help her sons become better people. She did what she could. They listened to her and understood there was a better way to treat people and do business. She was worried about her sons, but her husband knew the mountain roads and could handle himself. He would get everybody home safely. The rain was terrible.

On Election Day, conditions didn't improve. The sheriff and minister considered calling off the vote. They were both waiting for the rancher to arrive. He was due just before the voting started at 8 a.m... Shortly after 9:00, they decided to move forward with the vote without the rancher present. They did not know that outside of town the roads were much worse. Farmers and ranchers couldn't get to town. It rained all day. The sheriff decided at 5:00 that the election would be continued later when more people could vote. Most everyone agreed, even Dan and Thomas. These two men wanted it to be a fair election.

The storm cleared early on Sunday morning. By Monday afternoon, the rancher's wife rode to town to get the sheriff. The officer was wondering where the rancher was. He always came into town every couple of days, and no one had seen him since last Thursday. The wife explained that he was long overdue. The boys and their father had gone for some wood. They are probably fine but might need some help. The sheriff said that he would get a couple of men and ride out early tomorrow. The wife thanked him and rode home, fully expecting to see her family at home when she arrived. They weren't there. She was getting quite concerned.

On Tuesday around noon, the sheriff and his two helpers found the wagon down a deep ravine. It didn't look good for anyone in that wagon. The men yelled out, but there was no answer. They shot off a few rounds hoping to get a response. Nothing the sheriff would have to go back to town for more men, a big wagon, and some equipment that would allow them to look around down in the ravine and maybe retrieve anything down there.

The sheriff dropped by to tell the rancher's wife of their findings. The potential loss of her two sons was devastating. The sheriff asked if she had anywhere, she could go and wait. She explained that she really did not, but she would manage. She thanked him for going out to look today and was sorry that he had to go out again tomorrow. The response was that it is just part of the job. He gave her a quick hug and said good night.

The next day Dan and Sharon broke the news to Nancy. Dan had visited with the wife on several occasions over the years, and Sharon knew her. The women had visited many times and actually shared a few husband stories. The sheriff figured the news would be easier coming from someone she knew compared to a stranger like himself. It had been somewhat awkward the day before; she did not need that again. Dan and Sharon were comforting at a very difficult time.

Sharon said she was going to stay with Nancy overnight. Dan agreed and went back to town to finish some of the arrangements.

Sharon did the same things Nate had done for her. She held Nancy's hand, went for a walk, hugged her, and told her it is okay to cry as much as she wanted. The younger friend fixed Nancy dinner along with a stiff drink. Sharon explained the story of her husband's fall from the roof and how Thomas and Nate saved her from sadness and loneliness. Nancy talked about her boys. Both women cried.

Sharon told Nancy that it was going to be extremely difficult to move forward, but she had to persevere. Your friends will be a great comfort. She explained Thomas' loss. Nancy said that she now understood why such a nice man was starting anew in a strange town. She had met Thomas at church and visited once or twice while in town. Nancy told Sharon that she would probably go back to Chicago. Sharon kept Nancy talking while she drank one more drink. The drinks seemed to work, as Nancy was sound asleep within minutes of getting into bed. Sharon would fix any lingering effects of the alcohol in the morning. She had already handled that situation too many times in her life. Nancy was so glad that Sharon was there in the morning. She was very comforting.

Thomas and Nate came over about 10:00 to pay their respects. They were very respectful concerning the rancher and the boys. Thomas knew Nancy was not like her husband at all. He felt very sorry for her because a parent should not have to bury their children. He said as he touched her shoulder, "It might be out of place, but you have a very nice home." She thanked him. He asked, "What is your favorite part of the ranch?" Thomas was using Nate's strategy of keeping Nancy talking. Nancy showed them the kitchen and barn. Sharon had seen the kitchen the night before, expressing to Nancy how fantastic, it was. Now the two men, who knew their way around a kitchen somewhat, praised different aspects of the beautiful kitchen.

When the group walked into the barn, Nate went right to the horses. He went to each stall and whispered to the horse while putting his hand out. In no time Nate and all the horses were somewhat acquainted. Nancy commented that Nate must be special because the horses are not normally the friendly type. Thomas said that the horses sense Nate's kindness. Nancy stated that they each could use some of that as they have seen the whip excessively often. Nate told Nancy, "They are all beautifully configured, strong, and exceptionally good-looking except for the whip marks. I'd be willing to work with them to make them happier." Sharon chipped in that when Nate works with her every day, she is full of smiles and is very happy. Everybody enjoyed the humor.

"That's wonderful for both of you," said Nancy. "It would be great to see some smiles around here again. There used to be many years ago. As for the horses, I appreciate the offer, but that will be for the new owner to decide. I am selling the ranch. Once I get done with the business at hand, I'm moving back to Chicago."

"I think Dan can help you with the sale. He knows land prices and all the legal stuff. I think it will be a quick sale. It's the best ranch I've ever seen," said Thomas.

Nate asked, "Do you mind if we look around some? I have never seen such a stunning place. "

Nancy told the two men to make themselves at home. She and Sharon would go have a cup of tea and visit. Sharon enjoyed the tea and girls' talk. She had not done that since she was newly "married" years ago. The men thoroughly enjoyed their trip around the grounds. The blacksmithing area was top notch, the best of everything. Two windmills led to a couple of water tanks. One line went to the garden and barn area while the other went to the house. Nate had never seen a sawmill before. It was some distance away from everything, probably due to the noise. He really wanted to see it run. MAKING

YOUR OWN LUMBER WOW

"They have indoor water and a water supply for the stock and garden. Amazing," said the young man.

Thomas knew then that he was going to buy this place for Nate and Sharon as a wedding present. It would make M so happy.

Chapter 12
Doing Good Things

On Friday morning, the day before the extended Election Day, the four remaining members of the city council resigned and withdrew from the election. Word quickly spread around the town limits. Dan, Thomas, and the other three new members of the town council held a special meeting on Friday afternoon for anyone who could and wanted to come. Thomas and Dan did all the talking.

Thomas explained that the council had reviewed the books. It didn't appear that the monies received and paid out were very clear. The vet explained that there needed to be some other group of people to pay the bills of the town besides the council. Everything needs to be somewhat public knowledge. It should not be a secret how much comes in and goes out. The town council makes policy and decisions, allocates funds, and is in charge of raising money. The citizen group pays out the money through the local bank. All money received is recorded by the council and the citizen group and, subsequently, deposited in the bank. The town council serves the community. Its job is to listen to the people and then decide policy. This was the exact design M had developed when she was on the town council.

After the short meeting, the people in attendance clapped. Most suspected that the previous council was helping themselves to the town's money, but nobody wanted to challenge the sheriff and rancher. They were bullies and the minister wasn't far behind. There was no money in the small safe in the sheriff's office where the town's money was previously stored. This came as no surprise to anyone.

During the meeting, Dan gave a note to a local resident to deliver immediately to the minister. Another one went to the sheriff. After a couple of other clarifications of policy, the audience was dismissed as the council had some private business to attend to. They explained that it would be public knowledge rather quickly.

When the minister arrived, he didn't have the information that the council had asked for.

They wanted proof of his educational qualifications. When he couldn't produce any, he was told that his services were no longer required, effective immediately. The sheriff was called in next and told that this was his last month of employment in the town. He was rather upset and quit immediately. The council didn't say a word as he stomped out, but they were all smiling on the inside. He had used his position to impose unnecessary fines on people to pad the pockets of the town council.

Dan had talked to Colonel Jones when the officer came to the first town market about the possibility of hiring the military to patrol if a new town council was voted in. The newly elected town council would really appreciate the help. The Colonel loved the idea of helping the town. He also said that he had a sergeant who was retiring soon. The officer believed the retiree would be an extremely competent sheriff.

Thomas had filled in on a number of Sundays over the years as "acting minister". He was very knowledgeable, and his presentations were always noteworthy. Jeremy used to always comment, "The best minister in town is a vet". Thomas loved sharing his messages with the congregation. He and M had written the sermons together. He valued them so much, as did Marjorie, which he never threw them away. He had over a dozen and was ready to deliver them all. They were full of kindness, love, doing good deeds, and living a good Christian life. This was who the vet was.

The people heading to church were extremely surprised when they arrived on a nice bright sunny Sunday for the sermon. The doors of the church were open early with Dan outside explaining that the worshippers could enter and visit inside if they would like. Inside, the personable Dr. Smith welcomed as many as he could without pushing himself on them. He wanted to appear friendly but not overbearing. Nate and Sharon were both there saying their greetings to people. Nate was already making a name for himself with his fine artisanship. Sharon was known as a quiet woman who makes great jam.

After the sermon, one man started clapping. Soon the entire church was clapping. Dan had the biggest smile on his face. This town was changing. The man in front was leading the way.

On Saturday there had been four soldiers patrolling the streets with pistols furnished by Thomas and the Lieutenant. Dan's friend, Ed, was also carrying a pistol. There really was not a need for guns as this was a good town, maybe corrupt in terms of stealing money in the past, but there was never a problem with lawlessness on the streets. Dan still thought it was important to send a message. All five men also had the power to issue fines but were told by the town council to issue warnings first if appropriate.

Three men who said they would volunteer to be the three citizens to pay out the town's funds when appropriated by the town council approached Dan on Sunday. Dan thanked them and explained that it took two of them to sign for the money. He would add the sheriff to the list of signees as soon as one was hired. The lawyer added that the account would be set up on Monday. All three men were well-established members of the town. Nobody would argue about these three, as they were honest and hard working family men. By Sunday afternoon, several changes were in place, and things were off to a smooth start. Dan was thrilled that the town was moving in such a positive direction.

Thomas and Marjorie had discussed compliments over a period. They both agreed that these special words of praise develop immediate positive feelings and mood, build self-image, and motivate a person to move in a positive direction. Insults, on the other hand, pretty much did the opposite. Fake or phony compliments did not work either. A successful compliment needed to be genuine, given with some positive emotion and some enthusiasm. Thomas was amazed at how much Nate and Sharon complimented each other. He felt that they both loved giving more than receiving.

M had taught that compliments are a wonderful part of life. They motivate a person to do even better work in the future. People like to feel appreciated. Thomas knew that Sharon had grown up with virtually no compliments. Therefore, when Nate started giving her some compliments with the right ingredients, Sharon blossomed. Nate started filling her mind and heart with love, kindness, and affection. In very little time, Sharon let her emotions out. They had been kept in a bottle due to her situation in life. Accordingly, Sharon was able to give her Nate just the right type of compliments thoroughly enjoyed by the loving couple.

Seeing Sharon receive these wonderful words and actions from Nate allowed Thomas to completely understand M's lesson to him on compliments. She had said that it would be better for Nate to observe compliments given in his presence by his mentors. Marjorie thought that compliments come from the mind and, more importantly, the heart. Teachers can talk about expressing these kind words, but until the student develops the emotional side of a compliment, their words might manifest themselves in a cold, uncaring manner. A compliment delivered properly is a wonderful thing that has a dramatic positive effect. Now Thomas knew exactly why Nate had become an excellent giver of compliments to people. M had spent years teaching him about love, kindness, and affection, the emotional side of one is being that leads to the best types of compliments.

Thomas had an idea about the upcoming wedding. He wanted Sharon to wear one of Marjorie's dresses. He had kept the ones made by M's mother that were his and M's favorites. He would announce the request at dinner that night. The wedding was in seventeen days. He would talk to Dan tomorrow about the couple's wedding present. He knew that the newlyweds had Sharon's place, but he was very excited about the ranch. He didn't really know why.

Nate and Sharon fixed dinner as Thomas stayed away in the barn. He did have a few things to do, but the retired vet knew the young couple would enjoy their alone time better if he was some distance away. Yesterday the couple spent some time shopping in town. They mentioned that it was so much fun laughing and joking with so many friends about the wedding. They didn't appear nervous at all. The couple even checked the post office for mail. Nate gave Thomas a letter from his mother when they returned from shopping. It had come in on Friday afternoon.

The vet read it in the barn. He laughed, he cried, and felt extremely appreciated. He would keep this letter forever. He never realized that Mary gave all the credit for Nate's emotional growth to the Smiths. He is getting married to a wonderful woman because of the two best mentors in the world. She closed with the words, "I don't know who loves the Smiths more, Nate or M's little sister."

The dinner was great; Thomas loved being around the two "love birds". They had excitement and joy in their voices. Their smiles and laughs were contagious. The senior member of the group noticed that Nate and Sharon had never brought up mistakes made during their entire time doing chores. Thomas decided to ask the engaged couple if they had made some mistakes while working together. He wanted to hear Nate's answer. He personally liked not mentioning mistakes. They could change the mood. Did he want to risk it with Sharon present and wreck the mood at the table in front of his big question about the dress? He was very curious. Thomas figured he could fix the situation if need be. Anyway, he didn't think anything he did could change the couple's mood.

"Have you two made any mistakes as you have worked together?" asked Thomas. He smiled as he asked the question.

Nate answered, "Sharon and I are good workers, but we make a few now and then. We each made one last week. Sharon felt terrible when she made her mistake; I felt even worse. I explained to her what Marjorie taught me about mistakes. I also mentioned positive communication, another lesson from your wife, my second mother. Sharon and I decided that we would say only positive things after a mistake. In a few minutes, we would treat it like ancient history, known but never talked about. My favorite part of my mistake is when Sharon hugs me, kisses me, and tells me she loves me."

"That is a great way to handle mistakes," said a smiling vet. "It demonstrates so much kindness for each other. I love it."

Thomas explained that he had a big question he wanted to ask. Dinner was just about done, and Thomas figured he would show the couple the dresses. He would ask his pressing question and get back to dinner. Any dinner conversation would cover any awkwardness that might have arisen. He simply asked the couple to follow him for just a minute. Once the three entered the room, the dresses were hanging in plain sight. Thomas didn't even have to ask.

"YES, YES, YES!" exclaimed an emotional Sharon, "these dresses are absolutely magnificent. This is the best wedding present possible in so many ways." She hugged Thomas and then Nate. All three were very emotional.

The three spent the rest of dinner talking about the dresses and Marjorie. Thomas explained that Abigail, M's mother, made these dresses. She was very talented and extremely intelligent. Thomas mentioned that he was very fortunate that Abigail's daughter inherited her mother's brains and looks. Abigail taught Marjorie so much about life. Many of the lessons Nate learned from my wife originated with Abigail. These dresses were our favorites and only worn on special occasions. M would love that they found their way to you.

Before Thomas headed to town on Monday morning to see Dan about the rancher's property, he and Nate had a chance to talk in the barn while Sharon was finishing some things inside the house. Nate explained that he had never really seen so clearly the effects of kind words and small signs of affection on a person. Sharon has become such a kind person and so full of love and affection. All she needed were the right words, which he gladly provided. The happily engaged man quickly added that Sharon reminded him of M. Nate added that he was amazed by how many times he had used M's lessons when talking to Sharon. Thomas stated, "Sharon would pass these fine lessons on to others, just as you have, as she travels with you through life."

Dan completely explained the property to Thomas when his friend arrived at his office. He knew the vet was the only person in town who could afford the ranch. Dan had given the widow some numbers for the property late last week. Nancy quickly lowered them; she knew not many people could afford the ranch. The widow wanted a quick sale because she was ready to leave for Chicago. Nancy did think that the one person who could afford the ranch was Dr. Smith. There were a few rumors that he had some money.

Nancy liked the kind vet and knew he would involve Sharon and Nate in the running of the ranch. She really liked Sharon, a person who deserved so much more than she had been handed in her life. Her first impression of Nate was very positive. He seemed to really love Sharon. It showed in his actions when he was near her. The touching, the holding of hands, and his voice demonstrated strong feelings for Sharon. There was much talk about the couple. People really liked them together. It would give Nancy great pleasure to help Sharon and her person. The entire widow wanted was to live quietly with some old friends that she had kept in contact with over the years. She had no family left, so she had plenty of money.

Thomas found out from Dan that there were two employees on the ranch. They were hired to tend to a rather large herd of cattle. Nancy only asked that the next owner with an occasional day off better pay these men. Nancy told the lawyer that her husband treated the men as slaves. It was terrible. The men never left the old outbuilding far away from the house. They deserved better.

The price for the ranch was lower than Thomas expected. Dan pointed out that Nancy did not want to stay on the ranch or in town any longer than necessary. She had received some dirty looks from people. Nancy felt these were unfair but did not want to defend herself. She thought that people knew she had no control over her husband.

Dan told his vet friend that he didn't know about the cattle when he gave Nancy his appraisal of the ranch last week. After she told him about the beef, Dan said that he would ride out to determine their value. Nancy said that she wasn't concerned about a few dollars. Keep the price the same as they had previously agreed on. She just wanted to leave. Dan said that the ranch's price is a great deal for the buyer. Thomas told the lawyer to start the paperwork. He wanted to ride out and thank Nancy personally. Dan told his friend to hold off until the bill of sale is signed. There is no sense in getting too hasty. Thomas told his friend that he was completely correct. He was so excited about the sale that he had forgotten to cross his I has and dot his T's. Of course, he was smiling as he said these words.

Thursday morning Thomas went into town to discuss town council business with Dan. The lawyer was already paying Ed, but he wanted to come up with a number for the "sheriff" soldiers that would be fair to the army and to the town people. He also wanted the vet to know that he had ridden over on Wednesday to see Colonel Jones. "He introduced me to the retiring sergeant who is interested in becoming our town's sheriff. I believe the retiree will be great. He has a great presence and is very personable," explained Dan. Colonel Jones also knew what their town pays its sheriff and minister. Dan relayed the figures to Thomas.

The lawyer wanted Thomas to schedule a short town council meeting on Saturday afternoon to discuss these issues and anything else that might be of interest. He also handed the bill of sale papers for the ranch to Thomas to be signed. He had ridden out late yesterday afternoon to have Nancy sign. He mentioned that she was very pleased. Thomas thanked Dan for all the information on the ranch along with all his work on the bill of sale. He stated that he would stop by a council member's place who lived outside of town on his way to see Nancy. He would inform him of the meeting on Saturday and tell him not to worry about it if the meeting wasn't convenient for him. He would explain the agenda to let the member know what was happening in the meeting.

Thomas did not really like these short notices for council meetings. He thought that on Saturday's agenda there needed to be a discussion on an established town council meeting schedule. Maybe the time could even be agreed upon on Saturday. As he was leaving, Thomas mentioned that he would stop by the outpost to talk to the Lieutenant about the pay issue. Dan said he would contact the other two council members.

The personable vet went to the outpost first. The Lieutenant was very friendly. He congratulated Thomas and asked about the quality of work the soldiers were doing in town. The vet explained that everything was going very well. The soldiers are friendly and very attentive to the happenings on the street. The town council would like to compensate the men. The officer explained that wasn't necessary. The men are really enjoying the duty. Everyone thanks them for their help, making the men feel important. On most days, they receive a cookie or two along with some smiles from the young women. Everyday someone brings them sandwiches; at night, they get snacks and coffee. They really like that. It was finally agreed upon that the town council would donate to the soldiers' ration fund. As Thomas was leaving, he was thinking that this young officer was very good. He would tell Dan, hoping that it would get back to Colonel Jones.

The visit with Nancy went very well. Thomas thanked her several times during the course of their conversation. Nancy asked if Sharon and Nate were going to be involved in the operations of the ranch. Thomas smiled for a second and then said that he didn't know. Sometimes the owners of a property work the land; other times they lease it out. Nancy looked somewhat puzzled. The vet paused, smiled, and said, "It's my wedding present to the amazing couple."

Nancy was very happy that the ranch was going to Sharon and her fiancé. She told Thomas, "I've never seen Sharon so happy as on the day we had tea together while you and Nate looked around. I simply asked about her new person and Sharon went on for five minutes without stopping. She was smiling, full of emotion, and very excited about him. Sharon told me that she was sure that Nate loved her more than anything else on this earth, and she felt the same way towards him."

Towards the end of the conversation, Nancy excused herself for a second. When she came back, she was holding a bank bag with both hands. She explained that these coins are for the current town council to spend on the people. It is a small part of what the old town council stole from the town but please do not say where it came from. Nancy further explained, "I'm leaving on the early stage Saturday. I am so sorry for what my husband did, but I was no part of it. I tried to stop it at first but that did not end well for me. Please tell the town council that I wish them the best. Thomas, you seem like a very nice man."

Thomas told Nancy that he was going to take her to the stage. He would not take no for an answer. Therefore, it was agreed that he would pick her up at 7:30 a.m. The stage left at 8:00. Thomas realized on his way home that he would have to tell Nate and Sharon about the purchase. He was previously hoping to keep it secret until the three got home from the wedding. The secret was going to be impossible to keep with Nancy leaving. Her departure would be a major topic of discussion at the town market on Saturday. The news of Nancy's leaving would spread like wildfire, along with the identity of the buyer. He would tell the young couple at dinner.

The old vet was concerned that maybe he overstepped. Sharon already had her place. Both she and Nate were very happy with it. He was full of self-doubt all of a sudden. He questioned why he was so anxious to buy the ranch in the first place. He didn't normally operate in such a manner. Thomas was always well thought out and deliberate in his actions. This had always served him so well in his veterinary practice. All he could do now was to explain and hope for the best. He could always resell the property if need be.

At dinner, Thomas explained that he had done something big that involved both of his dinner partners. He apologized in advance for not asking them first. He told them to hear him out completely before they reacted. Then he dropped the news that he had purchased the ranch for them as a wedding present. The only reaction that he saw was Nate reaching over to take Sharon's hand.

Thomas explained to Sharon that Marjorie was very wealthy and wanted her money to be used to help people and do good things. That is why it did not bother him at all to buy the five acres and pay the materials to build and furnish the outpost. These were good things. The money spent on the town market was a great deed. Marjorie would have loved these things. She would have loved you two to have Nancy's ranch. M had a great sense of what would work. Her idea of a farmer's market was a huge success. That is why there is one here in this town now. She would have been thrilled at its popularity among the town folks.

Thomas stated that he believed that Marjorie was behind the purchase of the ranch. He always felt something whenever he saw the ranch. The kind mentor reminded his young protégé, "We don't do things in a rash fashion, but somehow I did, in fact, act quite impulsively." Thomas explained that he thinks M believes you two will do great things with Nancy's property. Thomas finished by saying, "I'm sorry if I overstepped. I surely did not intend to upset either of you. The purchase was completely done out of love by M and me."

Nate squeezed Sharon's hand three times, as he kissed her on the cheek. He nodded his head as he said, "Your comments are important to us."

Sharon was very surprised. She was thinking about Thomas' words the entire time. She figured out that the kind vet had not wanted to belittle her ranch at all. He was such a thoughtful and kind man. It was not in his nature to make fun of anything. In addition to this, my Nate just told me that my input is important. Both men seemed to be thinking of my feelings and me. She felt wonderful, wanted. Sharon spoke, "Thank you both for your words. Thomas, you bought the ranch because you followed your heart. I followed my heart when falling in love with Nate. I think we both made great decisions. I thank the Smiths so very much. I have always loved

Nancy's ranch. Nate, now we have two ranches that will become one, just like us."

Later, when the couple was alone, Sharon told Nate that ever since he opened her heart to his kindness, love, and affection, there have been times where she felt something. When they were at Nancy's ranch, she felt the sensation for a longer period. It was a warm feeling with a slight increase in her heartbeat.

Nate took Sharon in his arms and whispered, "It was Marjorie."

Sharon and Nate did chores in the morning on Friday and then went to town to buy flowers and candy for Nancy. They wanted to be there for her send-off. In the afternoon, they packed up the wagon with Nate's birdhouses and some firewood for the town market. The couple cooked dinner together. This was always such a good time. Nate thought this might always be his and Sharon's special time and place, much like M and Thomas' time in the garden. Again, he could not help thinking that so many things taught to him by M were things he used with Sharon.

On Saturday morning when Nancy and Thomas rolled up to the stage depot, Nate and

Sharon were there. Nate was holding some flowers and Sharon had a nice box of candy.

Sharon went first, "Nancy, you have been my friend for years when I had no one else. Thank you for that. You were always someone I valued. I am going to miss my good friend, but I will think pleasant thoughts about you quite often as I travel about on your amazing ranch." Sharon hugged her friend and kissed her on the cheek.

Nate handed Nancy the flowers while he said, "Nancy, thank you so much for what you did for us. You are a very kind woman with a beautiful smile. I hope you get to smile and laugh often in your new home." He also gave Nancy a hug.

Thomas hugged Nancy and whispered, "Thank you again. I guarantee that the newlyweds will do many good things with the ranch." He kissed her on the cheek.

As Nancy was getting ready to enter the stagecoach, three old acquaintances rounded the coach from the other side. They each hugged Nancy and said that they would have given her a small send-off party if they had known. The representative also said that everyone knows that nothing your husband did reflects on you. You are always kind and considerate. You are our friend.

Thomas helped Nancy onto the stage while Nate held her flowers and candy. After another quick goodbye and wave to everyone, the stagecoach started to roll. The widow really enjoyed the send-off; it was quite touching. Nancy sat there thinking that she had sold the ranch to a rather amazing and kind individual. If Nate was anything like Thomas, Sharon would love and be loved for the rest of her life. Nancy suddenly felt happier than she had been in a very long time.

As the stagecoach turned the corner and headed out of town, there were four women standing in the street with watery eyes, but Thomas quickly mentioned that today is town market day. He motioned for Nate and Sharon to hop aboard. Back at Thomas' place, the wagon was loaded and ready to go. A quick exchange from the buggy to the wagon, and the three were on their way. There had not been a market for three weeks, and Thomas was anxious to see the turnout. Nate and Sharon were going to sell biscuits and jam today. There would also be three birdhouses on the market. They were not sure how the biscuit sales were going to be received by the town folks, but Thomas stated that people do not expect you to continue handing out free biscuits and jam.

The Lieutenant handled all the preparations. Thomas was so impressed. This young officer was so organized and full of energy. He seemed to relish his role at the outpost. The people in town afforded Lt. Roger Haynes the utmost respect. He was a very pleasant, good-looking young man with a very friendly smile. He was rapidly becoming quite a VIP on the streets. He even patrolled occasionally with his men, but the officer always kept the correct military protocol. The men enjoyed the questions that the Lieutenant asked as it made them feel like he appreciated what they were doing.

The town market was packed. Many people came up to shake Thomas' hand, both for the election and the town market. Word had gotten around who had paid for the land and the materials to build the outpost. The same people were very impressed that the vet had volunteered to help build the structures. In a very short time, the people were realizing that Dr. Thomas Smith was quite a person. It was a great pleasure for him to see the market functioning to benefit the town. He bought a few items, but what he really liked was just enjoying the people without having to worry about trouble nearby.

A couple of acquaintances of the sheriff told Dan that the officer and the minister had moved a hundred miles to the west. The sheriff had family there, and there were jobs for both men. Dan relayed this information to his friend. Thomas was very relieved that these two had moved to a distant town. Both council members were very surprised that the sheriff and minister had been cowboys earlier in their lives.

Thomas talked to the local vet and explained to him that there were going to be many changes in town and beyond. The new everyday thoughts in this town were to do good things and be a positive influence. The new leader of the council also mentioned that the storeowner was already lowering all his prices. Thomas expected the vet to do the same. The owner of the store and the vet were not aggressive men. They had just been caught up with an aggressive rancher who wanted to be rich and powerful. Thomas was confident that both men would soon be doing the right thing.

Nate and Sharon were really enjoying everything about the day. Sharon was wearing her ring. It was a topic of discussion with every woman who came to the fire pit. The compliments and congratulations were nonstop. People loved the ring; everyone loved the wedding date. All the town market attendees seemed to really enjoy Nate and Sharon. They sold out shortly after noon and handed the fire pit over to a couple of soldiers who wanted to make cookies.

The happy couple headed over to their new place. Thomas said he would get a ride home with Dan. Sharon and Nate both wanted to check on the horses. Nancy also had an assortment of other farm animals: sheep, goats, chickens, and rabbits. There was ample food and water, but they all needed to be checked. Most of the time would be spent with the horses. The goal was to bring these horses to trust people again and, maybe, become friendlier.

Upon arrival, they each took one horse at a time to the outside coral where they walked and talked to each horse. The couple did this three times. The six horses were very glad to be outside. Nate brought the horses' food outside while Sharon was getting water. They didn't completely trust the horses, so they stayed pretty close to each other. The horses never approached Nate and Sharon, but they didn't shy away when approached. Nate figured this was a good first interaction with horses that had not been treated well.

They left the horses alone while they visited the garden, checked the other animals, and then took a tour of the house. Nancy had left everything! The furnishings were beautiful. The kitchen utensils and basement pantry food supplies were all there. The house was so large that Nate said that if they played hide and seek they would never find each other.

Sharon calmly stated, "Well, how would I hug and kiss my wonderful and amazing husband then."

Nate smiled and responded, "I like that word, my beautiful and talented wife. I will always whistle three times to bring you to me, especially if my heart starts to hurt." He whistled three times and Sharon gave him a big hug and kiss.

As the couple sat in the kitchen talking about the house, Sharon said that she wanted to give most of the canned goods away with Nancy's name attached to them. Nancy had given Sharon some tips on canning, so she knew the food was going to be fantastic. This would be a good thing in several ways. Nate took Sharon's hands, kissed them, and said that giving the goods away in Nancy's name is more than a great idea.

When the owners of the ranch left the house to get back to work, Sharon told Nate that she couldn't wait to teach him how to can food. It would be another fun thing they could do together. Nate squeezed her hand three times, as they reached the corals. The horses responded to Nate and Sharon in a more positive way when the couple took them back to their stalls. They both felt this was a great sign of things to come.

That evening at dinner, Thomas brought up the subject of chores. He had a plan. He laughed and said that he never did anything in haste. This brought out a smile from both of his dinner companions. The kind man thought that Nate and Sharon should take her horses to their new home. There were enough stalls inside the barn for all the horses and two corals outside. Dan was coming out to go on a ride with Thomas tomorrow. He was bringing a spare horse for the vet. "We will check on your stock, Sharon, as we ride through the countryside. Dan is really looking forward to it. He has not herded cattle since he was fourteen. We will also check your place over for you; it should be lots of fun. I will handle the chores at my place and your place from this point forward. Dan and I would love to help you herd your cattle to their new home. Thank you both for what you have done with the outpost and town market."

"Lieutenant Haynes wants to handle the town markets completely. He needs something to distinguish himself. The Colonel is coming in six weeks to fill out a fitness evaluation. The young officer is a very capable organizer. The town market is in great hands." Thomas finished up by saying, "I told Nancy that you two would ride out on Sunday to see the cattle after a quick visit to church to hear your favorite minister." He smiled.

Church was great. Nate has to hold Sharon's hand while they walked into church. She had a new dress courtesy of Nate who helped her pick it out on Friday while they were in town to get flowers and candy for Nancy. It was the best dress she had ever owned. Many people complimented her on how beautiful her dress was and how pretty she looked. Everyone noticed how happy she was. She smiled and laughed outside so much before church that some people thought Nate was tickling the hand he was holding. He was not; she was just that happy. During the memorable sermon by Thomas, at different times, Sharon and Nate squeezed each other's hand three times.

Sharon and Nate were simply shocked at the amount of land they owned. They were riding on a small road with flat land to the left, rolling hills to the right, and tree lined low rising mountains further to the right. Thomas had told them to keep riding on the road. It will veer to the right, and that is where the cowboys and cattle are. When the couple saw the number of cattle, they were simply astonished. Nate was shocked that there was fencing all around. He quickly opened the gate, and the couple rode into the pasture. Nate closed the gate because he didn't want any cattle escaping. He told Sharon that he didn't want to show off his cattle herding skills. They spotted the men and rode over to the cowboys.

Nate and Sharon introduced themselves to the two men. The two cowboys were very surprised that the rancher had sold the property because he loved cowboying. Sharon explained the whole story to the two men. The men were somewhat upset. It wasn't about the rancher and his sons; it was about their jobs. Sharon assured them that their jobs were safe. The lead cowboy thanked the new owners and mentioned that the previous owner and one of his sons always helped us move the herd. They are due to be moved to pasture three today. It is only about a mile away. The cattle know the way. It is a rather easy move.

Sharon spoke, "We can give you a hand. It would be our pleasure."

The four wranglers did move the cattle; it was an easy move. After the move, Sharon and Nate asked questions about pay, time off, and food rations. The two workers were thrilled with what Sharon said. All of a sudden, their quality of life increased dramatically. They had never seen a woman cowboy before. The hired hands were very impressed but maintained the utmost respect because she seemed to be the boss. Nate had told her riding out that she was completely in charge of what was to take place.

It was decided on Sunday's visit that on Wednesday, Sharon, four soldiers, and the two hired hands would drive twenty head to Colonel

Jones's town. Tim, the lead man, had informed Sharon that a shipment was due very soon. Sharon wanted to be there for the sale. She felt that the boss should know the procedure in such matters. She explained that Nate and Thomas or a couple of soldiers would watch the rest of the cattle. Tim explained that it was only nine miles to the fort. The whole trip takes about seven hours. Sharon was excited. She couldn't wait to see Colonel Jone's reaction to her being in charge. The four riders said their goodbyes, and the new owners of the ranch road back to the barn where they were going to be on horse detail for a while.

The couple spent three hours working with the horses. They both loved horses; it really wasn't work. They talked as they brushed, fed, and watered the horses. Time flew by. All of the horses were doing very well with each other. Sharon's horses had settled into their new home and were quite content after they were brushed. Nate and Sharon were also able to brush Nancy's horses. They too seemed to enjoy it. It was a very pleasant day. Nate mentioned to Sharon that in one week they'd be leaving to get married. Sharon stopped her work and walked over to Nate where she hugged and kissed him.

Nate finally said, "T, you make me the happiest man alive. Today has been so great seeing you handle the men and say so many kind things to them. They are going to enjoy having such a knowledgeable boss. I love watching you work with the horses, herd the cattle, and, most of all, I love just watching you."

For the next six days, everybody was busy. Nate started making horseshoes for the town in addition to working with the horses. In between blacksmithing work, he started on another birdhouse; each one was a different design. They were very popular at the market and always sold quickly. Sharon worked in the garden and tended to all the animals. The couple still handled the horses together. They were still staying at Thomas' place and looked forward to not having to make the round trip every day. Thomas was handling his and Sharon's garden. He loved the work. All day long, he thought about Nate and Sharon. At times, when he felt her, he talked to Marjorie.

He wasn't sad anymore. Thomas enjoyed talking about the man they had developed and the woman he was going to marry.

Nate took his breaks watching Sharon work. He praised her good work, got her a drink of water; always had a few smiles, maybe a joke and a laugh, and some kind words. It wasn't hard for Nate to do this. Words flowed out because Nate's heart was in charge. Sharon took her breaks watching Nate make horseshoes. She brought him water, some kind words, and many smiles. Her heart was also in charge.

Wednesday went extremely well. Sharon was a very capable boss but never offensive in any way. She asked questions about the drive, always wanting to know how things were done in the past. She thanked Tim often for his information. Mrs. Johnson knew two of the soldiers. They had worked on Sharon's ranch the day of the "big shooting match". Both privates enjoyed visiting with the boss and seemed to be really enjoying the cattle drive. The personable boss introduced herself to the two other soldiers and thanked them for helping. She also visited with Joe, the other hired hand, asked him a few questions, and, in general, made the men feel comfortable.

All the men realized early in the drive that Sharon knew what she was doing. She could really handle her horse. One question that Sharon asked Tim about was how many buyers were in town besides the army? She later used that particular information to negotiate a better price. She knew cattle. These were high quality and should bring top dollar. After the sale was completed, the two ranch hands asked if they could get a drink at the local saloon before heading back to the ranch.

Sharon explained very clearly, to the men, "There will be no drinking when you're on the job. I am sorry if that was allowed in the past, but, under my leadership, it would be negligent on my part to allow drinking. One drink can lead to two. That wouldn't work. You now have a day and a half off every week starting in two weeks from Saturday. This is when you are allowed to have a few drinks to relax. If you drink on the job, you will be fired. If you abuse alcohol when you are off duty, you will be warned once to reduce your drinking. A second offense will result in termination."

This was a big shock to both cowboys as the rancher had often brought out a bottle to share with his workers on his overnight stays. During the conversation on the way back to the pasture, the two hired hands were surprised to find out that Sharon got the best price ever for the cattle. The men always figured that the rancher was a top negotiator; they would have to rethink that. The cowboys also knew that in the past their drinking could be carried away at times. They could both make the change because they needed the jobs.

The benefits really outweighed the loss of a few drinks.

On Saturday, Sharon mentioned to Thomas that they had hired two soldiers to stay at the ranch. When the two soldiers arrived at the ranch on Friday for a briefing, they were given all the details. Sharon explained most of it to Thomas, "The major part of the briefing was the introduction to the horses. We do not want any setbacks in connection with Nancy's horses. Both men's main duty at the outpost is taking care of the horses. They are very good with the animals. One of the soldiers had asked if he could bring some small rounds of peppermint candy when he came for the briefing. I said it would be okay. I have heard of this friendly gesture from several people. Sure enough, Nancy's horses seemed to really like the peppermint candy. We feel relieved that the horses are in good hands." During the briefing one soldier asked me, "What's the name of the ranch?" "Luckily, we just happen to have one." Nate had stepped out just as Sharon was finishing. He showed Thomas the new sign that was to be hung at the entrance to the ranch. Thomas absolutely loved the sign.

He simply said, "Every day I am thrilled at what you two do together. Who designed it, if I may ask?"

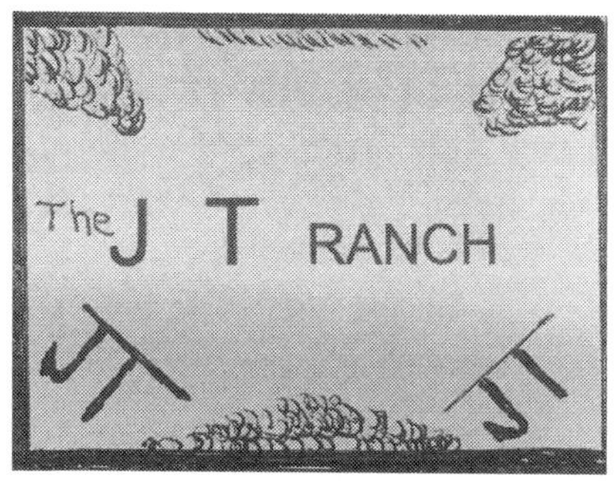

Nate answered, "It was Sharon's design. She helped me cut the wood. She burned parts of the sign as I made the brand for the cattle. The brand was also her design. We both made the letters of the ranch. She wanted each painted side except for the top to get bigger starting from the bottom right. Sharon thought it would be important to get the right start. Each painted side gets bigger to remind us that the ranch will continue to grow and prosper under our leadership. The sides are not perfect because my wife believes most things don't have to be perfect."

The vet finished the conversation by saying, "I love the sign. I will stop and think about your sign every time I see it. Sharon, thank you for your design and the thoughts behind it. Nate, I will enjoy the beauty of this sign – thank you."

Dinner was leftovers. They had packed everything beforehand for their early morning departure. The conversation at dinner centered on all the good work the three had done during the week. Towards the end of dinner, Thomas stated that he had thoroughly enjoyed the week in so many ways. It was going to be an early start, so the elder member of the group excused himself to get some rest. He thanked them in advance for cleaning up. He was not that tired but knew the couple enjoyed their together time doing dishes. Thomas was going to read a few letters from the past. He, like Marjorie, liked to revisit letters that had touched his heart. The first one was going to be Mary's last letter; it was such a special letter.

The next morning, the three left on time at 6 a.m. Dan was covering the sermon at church. He was excited about it. Thomas always loved the quiet early mornings. This one was quiet until they reached town. There were at least one hundred people cheering and clapping as the buggy went by. Sharon and Nate kept waving the entire time. The smiles never left their faces.

Thomas finally spoke as things quieted down, "I wondered why Dan asked me what time were we leaving; now I know. I told you that the town folks were going to love you two."

Chapter 13

the J T Ranch

The wedding was simply amazing. Jeremy had built a beautiful wedding arch. Mary decorated the arch and various places surrounding the ceremony with flowers and greenery. She also decorated the main aisle. Thomas walked Sharon down the aisle as the music played. Nobody was sitting. Andy, Doris, Nate, and Jeremy were gathered under the arch with Jack, Mabel, and Mary standing very close by. Yesterday, Jeremy explained to Nate and Sharon what was going to transpire next. He did not want to overwhelm the couple with what Mary had designed to happen after Thomas and the bride reached the arch. Once Sharon took her spot, Jeremy asked everyone to join hands. It was pretty much a circle. Jeremy explained that this family was a gift from God. It was full of love and kindness with each member supporting each other. He welcomed Sharon into the family and thanked her for being so kind, loving, and supportive. He mentioned that Sharon's new clan adores her smiles and laughs. "We are all so blessed to have this family," said the very happy minister. He then told everybody to go back to their spots.

The ceremony itself was short, but it was very emotional for everybody. Sharon was maybe the happiest of all. The other eight attendees told her that she was beautiful and looked stunning. Even Andy complimented the bride, and he didn't even like girls yet.

Back at the house, everybody enjoyed visiting. Sharon noticed that Mabel was starting to show. They had an enjoyable conversation where the bride congratulated Mabel on her remarkable garden. Sharon also mentioned that she and Nate were so happy about the forthcoming addition to the Brown family. Sharon thanked Jack, while visiting with him, for teaching Nate such wonderful skills. During the conversation, she could clearly see that Jack was a kind and loving man. He seemed like the perfect mentor. He was definitely going to be a great dad. He also seemed to be a humble man who possessed great skills and strength. She really liked that. She knew

Jeremy, Doris, and Andy from her previous visit. She enjoyed talking with all three, but the person who really impressed her was Mary. They had, of course, visited before, but since yesterday Mary had become even kinder with more hugs and touches. She also displayed that warm wonderful smile quite often. Mary told Sharon that she could call her Mary, M2, or Mom, whichever she preferred.

When Mary approached the bride after arriving back at the house, she gave her a big, long hug. Mary took Sharon's hand, led her away from everybody, and told her that we need some privacy for a minute. M2 took Sharon's other hand and, while holding both firmly, spoke slowly, "You are perfect for my son. He loves your looks, smiles and laughs, but, more importantly, he admires what you do, and really adores who you are. His love for you knows no bounds. He will demonstrate that love each day. I have known him for his entire life (she smiled and squeezed the bride's hands). I have never seen him happier. He lights up when he is talking about you. He knows about love because Marjorie taught him. He always wondered about the ultimate love of a spouse. Then he found you and knew firsthand what M had been explaining to him. Thank you for making my boy the happiest man on earth. You both are truly blessed to have each other."

Sharon replied that she felt the same way about Nate. Both women were actually crying some. Nate walked over to where his mother and Sharon were standing. He was curious about the tears. His mother explained, "Women cry sometimes when they're extremely happy, and Sharon and I have never been happier in our entire lives."

"Me too," said Nate. The three group hugged.

Mary eventually gravitated towards Thomas. They drifted off from the group to have a private conversation. Mary explained to this dear man that when she talks to M nowadays, she is not sad. M2 stated that she does not understand it, but she is always happy after the talk. Mary told Thomas that one day she told his wife that she could only hope that there was a window in heaven, so M could see the man she created achieve such wonderful things. Today would be one of those days. She asked Thomas if he felt her here today.

Thomas said, "Yes, she was here. When I came out of the church, I walked over to a tree that Marjorie always loved. There was a light beam hitting the trunk. We had witnessed this before, but today as I neared the tree, the beam seemed to get brighter. I felt very warm; I knew she wanted me to know that she was there. There was no doubt in my mind that she had seen everything. In a few seconds, a cloud covered the trunk, and I cooled down. I think her work on earth may be done. I, like you, am no longer sad when I talk to her. I am meeting new people in the town where I live, I have work, and I have Nate and Sharon. They bring me great joy. I'm convinced I will get to witness a few of the great things they will do together."

Early the next morning, the clan gathered for an early breakfast before the three travelers got on their way. Nate spoke for an extended time. He thanked his mother and father for the perfect wedding. He and Sharon loved everything about it. He told Jack, Mabel, and Thomas how special they were to him. The newly married man continued to speak, "The Johnsons were more than blessed when the Smiths and Browns entered our lives. Sharon and I thank Jack and Mabel for the cabin and Mabel for decorating it so wonderfully." He went to his sister and brother, hugged them, and said, "Sharon and I want to thank you for being part of our wedding. The memory of you standing next to us during the ceremony is something we will cherish forever." Nate mentioned Thomas in his closing statement. He finished with the words, "Thomas, bless you for bringing Sharon into my life; she is perfect. My lessons from the Smiths are now complete. Each of you gets an A+." He smiled.

Sharon stood up and said, "Thank you all for welcoming me into your family. I have never met such wonderful people. We loved everything about the wedding. Thank you so much, Jeremy and Mary. Thomas told me awhile back that I was going to meet some great people. He was right. I will always do my best to be as loving and kind as you all have demonstrated to me."

As Sharon was wiping away tears and sitting down, a buggy pulled up carrying a man and a woman. The man said that they were sorry to interrupt; please don't get up. He read from a piece of paper that he and his wife just came by to give Sharon and Nate a wedding present from the town. All the town folks have seen this talented and marvelous man grow up. He is family to us. Everybody hears that Sharon is simply amazing, so the town welcomes her as an honorary member. Without further ado, here is some startup money for your wonderful journey together.

Nate jumped up, shook the man's hand, thanked him, and told him to thank the whole town. Nobody in the Johnson clan knew the couple that rode up. The town had planned it that way, to not take up too much time. They knew the goodbyes at the Johnson house would take quite a while. They did.

Thomas was driving the buggy out of town. There was some small talk, but before long,

Nate and Sharon were asleep. They slept off and on for three hours. They woke up when Thomas stopped to take the horses to a small nearby pond for water. Nate took over the reins, and the three talked about everybody at the wedding. It was very enjoyable. Sharon learned more about Doris and Andy. Mabel was doing very well. Jack was busy with work and had never been as happy as he was now. Mary had been asked by the town council to please attend meetings. They wanted her to replace a member who was stepping down. There was no doubt that she would be voted in.

The travelers arrived home Saturday around 10 a.m. They were all glad to get home. Thomas said that he was going to take a quick nap. Nate and Sharon took the buggy out to the JT ranch. The newlyweds were glad to be at their new home. The soldiers met them in the yard where they had been working with the horses. They explained that they had a very pleasant experience. The men mentioned the many things that were done, but Sharon and Nate remembered only one thing. The horses did very well. The soldiers even rode all ten. They did mention that the army horses and Sharon's horses have to be quite friendly. The two young men thanked Sharon for the job and said they would be happy to "babysit" anytime. Everyone seemed happy with the work that was accomplished during the week.

Nate and Sharon put on their work clothes and decided to go on a ride to see the cowboys. After a short visit, they just might explore further to the south to see what the land looked like. It was very exciting to own so much land. Nate always had some extra money as he grew up. He were paid from the Smiths and received a small amount from Jack and his father from time to time. Sharon, on the other hand, never had any money growing up. After getting married, any money she received from her canned goods sale always went towards food. Her husband always kept the money from any sales he was involved with. Now Sharon felt so rich in so many ways.

The hired hands explained that everything was fine. They did ask if Nate and Sharon could help them move the herd. The task was quickly accomplished with the bride quietly complimenting Nate on his newfound skill. The boss told the hired hands that they would be off duty from 6 p.m. on Friday until 6 a.m. on Sunday. They would be paid on Friday when they reached the ranch. There were beds in the barn, a fire pit for their use, and a washbasin. She would explain in more detail when they arrived on Friday. The men thanked her for her kindness. They also mentioned that she really knew how to cowboy. She silently nodded her head while touching her hand to the brim of her cowboy hat. The boss and her man turned to start their adventure of exploring the ranch.

As the newlyweds started out, Nate said, "The hired hands really like their new boss, respect her, and appreciate all her skills. You have made their lives so much better." He continued to say, "I love seeing my wife do good things. You do it so naturally without any gruffness. You use kindness with some smiles. Your knowledge and intelligence shines forth. You remind me so much of a friend of mine, maybe you're heard of him, a Dr.

Thomas Smith."

Sharon put her arm out, signaling for Nate's hand. He provided it. She squeezed it for about five seconds before letting go. She thanked him for such a meaningful compliment. She had watery eyes. The bride explained that nobody has ever valued me as if you do. As soon as we stop, you just might receive a token of my appreciation.

Nate quickly reacted, "I think my horse picked up a rock. Can you help me dislodge it?"

Sharon laughed and said, "Nice try, but your horse is just fine. Be patient, my darling. I can't give out too many hugs and kisses; they might get old."

"Oh, my lovely wife," said a smiling Nate, "your affection never gets old. I need it because it fuels my heart."

The couple loved the scenery. They even came across a small pond fed by a spring while they were riding up a canyon. Sharon was carrying her pistol and had one of Thomas' rifles holstered in a fine leather scabbard attached to the saddle. Sharon had not taken her pistol out of her dresser in many years. She liked having it with her. As the couple rode on towards the end of the property, two things came into sight almost simultaneously: a property sign became visible saying in big letters, PRIVATE PROPERTY NO TRESPASSING and a slight distance away a herd of beautiful wild horses.

Nate asked Sharon, "Do you think they can read the sign?"

His wife calmly said that she did not know because she hadn't met them yet. She mentioned that the two on the left are too young for school, but that big person on the right looks like he has been "schooled" many times. They certainly are a pretty bunch of horses. Nate concurred as he dismounted and slowly started walking towards the herd; Sharon joined him. She had a few apples with her. They also had their horse's right beside them. The couple didn't want to get too close; this was just an introduction. They stood about one hundred yards away petting their horses, not looking at the wild herd. Sharon then slowly took five steps towards the herd and put the apples down. The ranchers slowly mounted their horses and eased away from the herd.

The newlyweds stopped under a large tree, so the horses could rest for a few minutes. Each person felt so lucky to be in the presence of the other. Nate loved Sharon's looks, mannerisms, smiles and laughs, and her love for him showing on her face, in her expressions, and in her words. Sharon loved Nate's words, his kindness and thoughtfulness, and his total love for her. The more he showed these things, the more she loved him. The more she showed her love in her actions, the more Nate loved her. After Nate picked up some fuel for his heart, he was thinking about the compliments Sharon had given the soldiers. It rather reminded him of M. Sharon was becoming someone quite special, and she was his wife. WOW!

About halfway home, Sharon asked Nate if she could buy some undergarments. He replied that he had been thinking about money lately. He wanted to share his thoughts and get Sharon's input on the matter. He mentioned that he liked the thought of having two "jars". One would hold spending money; the other contained ranch money. The loving husband asked his wife what her thoughts on the matter were...

Sharon replied, "I've never had any money, so I don't have any experience in saving. I find it very exciting to have some extra money. I'll trust what you say."

Nate explained, "The money in the jars is very flexible. If the ranch money gets too small, we can always move some money. We don't have yours and mine money. It is our money. You may take it all if you want something. I would gladly agree with whatever you do. If buying something makes you happy, then I'm happy." "J, I love you so much," said a watery-eyed Sharon.

The young couple fixed dinner for themselves and Thomas. He rode a borrowed horse out to the JT and would drive the buggy back with the horse attached. He was going to review his notes and words on the sermon with the newlyweds; Nate and Sharon enjoyed the preview. Thomas had such a gift. It wasn't just the words he spoke, but the style and emotion always touched whoever heard the words. Sharon believed that Thomas would be the minister for the town as long as he wanted to be. He was that good.

Everything about the Sunday sermon was excellent. The people enjoyed entering the church early to visit. Smiles, laughter, and friendliness filled the air. The minister loved the change in the congregation. The town people were starting to really enjoy each other. Thomas knew this Sunday behavior would soon become the normal way individuals interacted throughout the week. Everybody loved Thomas' words. The town was responding quickly to his teachings.

Thomas cut the sermon short by five minutes to mention a civic topic. He apologized for cutting the sermon short but needed to speak about Nancy. "Most of you know that she was a kind lady. Nancy left a substantial amount of canned goods for those who might need a helping hand this winter. The town council, with input from all of you, will decide how the distribution will happen. In addition, two weeks from this coming Saturday, Nancy will be sponsoring a dinner and dance right after the town market. It is free for everybody thanks to Nancy. I only wish that Nancy were here to continue spreading good deeds, along with providing a kind and positive attitude. When I moved here from my old town, many people sent me a number of letters. I enjoyed the stories of their daily lives as I had lived there for so long. These folks were my friends. Next Sunday I will have a large envelope with Nancy's current address. If you like, you can drop a letter in the envelope. I will mail it on Tuesday."

The gifted and talented minister spent the rest of the day at Nate and Sharon's place. There were a variety of subjects discussed, mixed in with many laughs and smiles. Sharon never got tired of the friendly and positive atmosphere. The smiles and laughter came easily around these two men. Sharon had never initiated much humor in her life, but she was catching on quickly. She was starting to contribute more and more to the humor. It helped being in the presence of these two connected kindred spirits. She watched, listened, and learned. Nate started to notice Sharon's humor. It was very much like the wit that he had learned from Thomas and Marjorie. Sometimes she was just silly or cute, sometimes it was directed at herself, but it was never meant to embarrass or hurt anybody. Nate really liked that.

Thomas asked the married couple if they could do him a favor. Sharon jumped right in with the words, "Well, Thomas, I've only known you for a short time, but I've been keeping track of how many favors I owe you. I think it is 137. The town record is 151. I don't know what to do. Do I help you go for the record, or do you a favor. I'll have to ask my very smart husband." She was smiling almost the entire time with a twinkle in her eye. The men loved it.

"My mother would be the person to talk to," said Nate. "She has a great mind for numbers, but I think she would say favors are never counted, only flavors matter, especially in cookies and pies."

"Let's go bake some cookies," responded a laughing Thomas.

As the three headed for the house, Thomas commented, "All three of us got a good laugh out of the word favor. You two are special. By the way, you would be doing me a huge favor by taking the wagon. I don't need it any longer as my vet days are over. I would love to see it put to use at the JT Ranch."

Sharon loved those words "doing me a huge favor by taking the wagon". You could give someone something using those words. They would probably think they were helping you out. Many people would not take anything from anybody. They felt like it was charity. Charity is for the poor. Sharon's dad was a prime example. He never accepted anything from anybody, and they were definitely poor. She was going to remember those words from Thomas.

The three chefs made some of Sharon's special sugar cookies. They, of course, had to sample them. The smiles and laughs continued as they ate half the cookies. Sharon had made a stew right after getting home from church. It was still slow cooking on the top of the stove. She started preparing biscuits as the men went back outside to talk. Thomas had a few things that he wanted to discuss with Nate.

Thomas mentioned that he was very aware Nate did not like killing any animals. The vet continued that he could dress out the chickens and rabbits. He had done that hundreds of times for M. He would be glad to do it for Sharon. The retired vet also told Nate he and Dan had gone up a canyon that just happened to lead them to the wreck where Nancy's family was lost. There is some good lumber and many parts of the wagon that are very salvageable. I would be more than willing to help you recover anything you think is worth the effort.

Nate thanked his mentor for both offers. He thought he had better learn to dress out the small animals. Maybe Sharon might want to learn also, but he doubted it, as she was more of an animal lover than he was. Nate asked if Thursday was a good day to go up the canyon. Thomas replied that 9 a.m. on Thursday would be great.

Nate had already resolved in his mind that living in Sharon's old house was okay. He figured that his life with Sharon started a short time ago. His life with Sharon would definitely be his focus. It was all that mattered. Once again, Thomas spoke some words to Nate that made perfect sense. The kind man explained that Sharon was like something that had been stepped on and pushed down into the mud. It couldn't breathe the air or shine in the sun. You picked up the object, cleaned it off, and found a bright wonderful diamond. Sharon is a joy to everyone, but she was able to find you. You found her. Her love and devotion exploded outward as she had met her perfect match. You found your perfect match. Seeing you, two together is a beautiful thing to watch.

Their time together, although short, had been magical. He agreed that Sharon was a perfect match for him. The two newlyweds valued each other in so many ways. It was all that really mattered. Marjorie had taught that yesterday was gone; it can't be changed. Focus on making today a good day; hope and plan to make tomorrow a better day. Never dwell in the past; life goes on. Nate had already learned that lesson. Getting materials from the canyon was going to be easy. He would not even think about the rancher and what happened. He would keep moving forward.

Dinner, as usual, was very pleasant. The conversation was nonstop. Thomas asked a multitude of questions about the ranch. The friends shared any knowledge that might be of benefit to the others. Interesting points of view about the town and its future direction were of particular interest to Sharon. Nate had some very intriguing ideas about it. She was very surprised. Thomas was an expert in planning and financing town projects. He was very excited to get started on a town square. During the various topics of discussion, everyone enjoyed Sharon's stew and biscuits. Both were very tasty. She admitted that she had followed one of Nancy's recipes. Thomas quickly asked if he could have the recipe.

Sharon responded, "I can see that you are following Mary's advice. Flavors are to be enjoyed. Flavors really count. Favors, on the other hand, should never be counted, 136. I will copy it down and give you a copy as soon as Nate and I finish the dishes." The men loved Sharon's smile when she said 136. Humor is so great.

Thomas thanked the skillful cook for the great dinner and the recipe. Nate explained to the vet, "Sharon and I want you to spend the night a couple of times a week. There are many chores to do, cookies to bake and eat, and horses to groom. We also have six riding horses. The three of us could go for an afternoon ride. It would be great having you out for a few days at a time." Thomas thanked both of his hosts and said that coming for a couple of days sounds like fun. The vet did like to keep busy. It was decided that he would come out Wednesday morning with the wagon and spend the night.

Monday and Tuesday were identical days. The newlyweds worked together on some things like the garden and the horses, and apart on other things like blacksmithing and cleaning the house to get ready for Thomas' arrival. On Tuesday afternoon, Sharon surprised Nate when she said to him that she wanted to help build the birdhouse. Nate loved it.

The romance between the two carried on throughout the two days. They both loved Thomas, but being alone made these days very special. Nate had always enjoyed his time with Marjorie, but the time with Sharon was even better. M had been so right about the connection between spouses. The communication, both spoken and unspoken, highlighted each day. They each loved showing the other their work. The compliments flowed easily between the two. Each person's very essence was enhanced because the compliments were perfect; the right words were spoken with just the right amount of enthusiasm and love.

By the time dinner preparations were started on both nights, the spoken words dwindled, but the touching and kissing increased substantially. Nate loved this time, doing work that you enjoy, watching the one you love working, and sharing the moments together. Sharon enjoyed it even more. This was the first time that she felt truly connected to someone.

On Wednesday morning, Sharon headed to town in the buggy. She had money in her pocket for the first time and was going to spend it on some items that she liked. She was in a splendid mood. After pulling the buggy to a stop, the new bride saw two little girls who she estimated to be about four and seven. She greeted them and noticed the little one was somewhat sad. Mrs. Johnson asked if everything was okay. The older sister responded that her sister wanted to go see the horses at the livery stable, but their daddy said no. Sharon explained that you should always do what your parents say. The older sister said that their mother died.

"I'm so sorry," Sharon said as the girls' dad walked up. "Hello, I'm Mrs. Johnson. You have two very cute daughters."

The man answered, "How do you do? My name is John Jacobs. My tall one is

Elizabeth and my short one is Ruthie. Have they been bothering you, Mrs. Johnson?"

Sharon explained that they were absolutely no bother at all. She mentioned they might even share a love of horses. She asked John if he had been in town for a while because she had been here for ten years and had never seen him before. It is always a pleasure meeting new acquaintances. Mr. Jacobs stated that they do not get to town very often and drop in occasionally for a few supplies. Now it is back to work. He also mentioned that they have been in town for about three years.

"Well, it was certainly nice to meet you all, John, Elizabeth, and Ruthie. I have made three new friends today. I think that is great," said a smiling Sharon. She was so personable. As usual, the friendly new bride made quite an impression on all three, especially the girls.

Sharon had a great time in town while shopping. She knew that her entire demeanor had changed since meeting Nate and Thomas. It was as if someone had opened a box and out jumped a smiling, witty, and charming new person. Everybody she greeted as she walked through town saw this transformation. The people were so happy for her because they knew of her prior situation. The amazing thing was that Sharon didn't have to think about being friendly; it just came out. When she introduced herself to the clerk in the clothing store, it was as if they were instant friends. Again, Sharon smiled as she introduced herself as Mrs. Johnson. She felt so happy saying those words.

Before leaving town, she dropped by to see Dan for a minute. He wasn't busy with anyone as she walked in. He welcomed her into his office and asked if she would like to sit and have a soda. Sharon thanked him for the offer but declined as she flashed that contagious smile. She did say that she had a question for him. She explained that she had just met John Jacobs and his daughters. "Do you know them?"

Dan explained that John's wife died last year. He is a very proud man and will not take any help. He has been struggling to work and take care of the girls. He looks tired and stressed over the whole situation, but he perseveres. He is a good man. He makes extra money selling firewood to the people in town. On top of all the work raising two little girls by himself, his horse up and died three months ago. Thomas is aware of the situation and plans to help John in some way.

As soon as Sharon arrived back at the JT Ranch, she saw Thomas and Nate working with the horses. They had saddled two of Nancy's horses and were walking them around. She quickly asked if they were going to ride the horses today. Thomas replied that they weren't sure but were thinking about it. Sharon rushed into the house to change clothes. She figured that she should be the first one to ride one of Nancy's horses. She was a very good rider and had a great calming effect on horses. She definitely didn't want Thomas to be the first one aboard one of the horses. These horses were an unknown to the new owners as far as riding was concerned. If someone was to be thrown, let it not be Thomas.

When Sharon left the house, the men were still walking the horses. Sharon asked if they thought the horses were ready to ride. Thomas replied that he thought his horse was definitely ready. Sharon asked if she could be the one to ride him. The best rider explained that she has worked with this horse extensively. Sharon mounted the horse and left the corral. She rode for about ten minutes and then returned to the corral. She told the men that this horse was top quality, strong, smooth, and very responsive.

"Nate, do you mind if I take your horse for a small ride?" Asked his smiling bride.

"That would be great but hurry back. I want to hear all about your trip to town," said an interested husband. "I'll start to cool down your horse and start to brush him out as you become friends with your next mount."

"Thank you, I'll hurry with this horse. My hand got a chill on my last ride and needs to be held for a few minutes," said Sharon as she winked her eye towards the people.

When Sharon returned, Thomas stated that he would take care of the horse. He asked them to start preparing a small lunch. He was thinking that he would give them at least thirty minutes to finish the task. He never wanted to infringe on their private time. Thomas remembered how much he enjoyed his time with Marjorie. This young couple valued "their time" just as much as the Smiths did. HOW WONDERFUL FOR THEM The vet stated that when he comes in for lunch he'd need a full report on the second horse. It appeared to the expert horse vet that the four riding horses Nancy left behind were excellent riding stock. He could personally attest to their health. They were magnificent.

Thomas watched the couple walk hand in hand towards the house. He never got tired of seeing the affection between the two. It warmed his heart every time. He also took note of what Sharon had just done. She asked to ride the big, strong, strange horse under the pretense that she knew him so well. The vet knew she was just protecting him. She was, by far, the best rider of the three. Every day as he saw Sharon do things, he became more impressed with the person he had introduced to Nate. She had many of the same mannerisms as M, along with many skills she had developed in her journey through life. Nate was the recipient of all of this, plus a devotion and love from Sharon that was stronger than anything Thomas had ever seen.

Several topics of conversation during lunch were different from the normal banter. Nate explained to Thomas, "Sharon and I would love for you to have one of Nancy's horses. We already have our two riding horses that we are very comfortable with." The proud husband smiled as he mentioned, "I think my beautiful wife might be the best cowboy in town. She and Rusty are quite a pair. I get jealous." As Nate continued to speak, Sharon grabbed his hand and squeezed it three times, "Nancy left four riding horses and two work horses. You can have your choice. You can stable it here or at your place; whatever is more convenient for you." Thomas thanked them. He thought he knew the horse he would take. The vet said that he would talk to the horse to see if it was okay. He returned Sharon's wink from earlier that day.

Sharon discussed her new friends with Nate and Thomas. She explained John's situation. She asked Nate and Thomas if helping the Jacob's family was a possibility. Both men were immediately supportive of the idea. Sharon explained that she had a plan. It was not dishonest or anything like that. It would start out as a friendly gesture and build into a friendship that would allow us to befriend the entire family. She laughed and said that she always wanted to be an aunt.

Now it was Thomas' turn to mention something that he hoped would be okay with Sharon.

He purposely waited until lunch was finished before bringing up the subject. He informed the married couple that he was going to fix dinner, and rabbit was being served. He quickly pointed out that if this is uncomfortable for you, Sharon, the menu can be changed. Sharon responded that she had eaten rabbit many times but never one that she fed and cared for.

She smiled, took Nate's hand, and stated that it is time to face the reality of life. She took Thomas' hand with her other hand and thanked him for helping us move in the right direction. Nate remembered Marjorie smiling and doing the same thing one day with her hands as she had thanked Nate for such a great day. UNBELIEVABLE

Dinner was fun with many smiles and laughs as part of the conversation. Nate had observed the rabbit preparation very carefully. He mentioned to Thomas that he would do the next one with his mentor watching, just like old times. Thomas enjoyed that comment beyond words. He had grown to really value what he had done for Nate. Towards the end of dinner, Sharon explained her plan regarding John Jacobs. Both men thought it was a very personable design. Thomas believed that it was a style that M would have thought of. Very Impressive

"You have a gift with people that allows you to become friends almost immediately. I'm excited that we will become friends with the Jacobs," said a smiling Nate. "I'm really looking forward to meeting Elizabeth and Ruthie. It should be lots of fun. You can mentor the girls while John helps me with chores. I think we can use some help around here, especially if we start running the lumber mill."

The men left early Thursday morning in the wagon. While Thomas was hitching up the horses to the wagon, Nate explained to Sharon that they would be gone for quite a while. They were going to salvage some items that might come in handy. He gave his wife a big hug, a long kiss, and some touching romantic words. Sharon responded in a like fashion. Thomas saw some of this going on. He knew that Nate was anxious to get going, but he was not going to rush off as if many husbands do. Nate had his priorities in order, so wonderful for the newlyweds.

Chapter 14

More Good Deeds

There were a number of interesting events over a short period of time that would set Thomas and the Johnsons on a course that would occupy much of their energy for the next two years. The three, along with Dan, were paramount in setting the tone for the town. Sharon spearheaded the town store and food bank that was located in the building that had been previously used to sell homemade goods to benefit the town council. She turned it into a community project for the women of the town. Inside the store, there was so much positive energy and such a good feeling of doing something wonderful. Sharon had a dozen women involved; the wives loved to help. They all enjoyed their new spokesperson and leader, Sharon Johnson. Many men, although busy with their own lives, were also impressed by Sharon's words at town council meetings. She spoke often about town projects or any concerns the people might have. People liked her thoughts.

Dan and Thomas worked on the town council for two years. In that time, they raised money for a splendid town square. It was a meeting place for many people in town. They would visit with friends and meet new ones. There was a small bakery right next to the square run by a local restaurant; it was designed to be a nonprofit. This kept prices very low. Many days, towards the end of the bakery's day, the workers gave away anything they had leftover. The bakery was the design of Thomas and Dan. Both men often praised the restaurant publicly. They explained how fantastic it was that the restaurant was benefitting the town. They were to be commended because, in this instance, they were placing good deeds over profits. The restaurant was making the town a better place.

Thomas led the change in taxing local stores. Previously, all stores within the town limits paid tax. The ranches and farms outside of town paid none. The new town council felt this was unfair. Many of the people outside of town could easily afford to pay some sort of tax to support the town, whereas many stores in town barely made any profit. The citizens decided to hold fundraisers for specific projects like the town square. No taxes were to be levied by the town council. The town dinner and dance were the primary fundraiser for the town; they were very popular.

Since there were no secret dealings within the new town council, the town actually knew the balance of the town's money. If there were a need for money, the town council, the three-person committee, and the sheriff would schedule a donation day for the town. All donations were anonymous. People would give because it was the right thing to do.

Thomas always thanked the donors after one of his touching sermons, and he would mention it again at the next town dance and dinner. Nate thought the vet's words sounded so much like Marjorie's. They were moving and inspirational.

The town council expanded the school from one room to three. The town hired one more teacher, making it a total of two for the town. These teachers handled the lower grades while Dan, Thomas, and a local woman named Betty with college experience handled the older students. Dan had explained earlier that much of the older students' work was done independently. The three mentors could monitor and assist when necessary. Thomas loved being there to assist and teach a lesson now and then. Teaching and preaching occupied much of his time. He really enjoyed sharing his knowledge. Everybody who encountered Dr. Smith learned to appreciate this kind and knowledgeable man. His smile was still very contagious.

Nate wasn't in charge of any project in town. He loved helping in any way possible. The lumber mill had been up and running during most of these two years. John Jacobs and Tom Moore were the ones working the mill. Nate was in charge, but both men were very capable. It was more of a team effort than anything else was. Any lumber needs of the town were now produced locally at a very reasonable price. Nate supported Dan, Thomas, and Sharon in their work. He especially loved supporting and helping his wife; she always responded affectionately. Every day Nate felt very satisfied that, he was doing good deeds. He would occasionally hear the words of Marjorie as he went through his day. At night when he and Sharon shared their positive stories of the day, she would take Nate's hand and smile as he was talking. He felt truly blessed. His wife was doing good things. She had become his Marjorie and much more.

Sharon's plan to incorporate the Jacobs family as friends of the Johnsons and Dr. Smith worked to perfection. After a stop by visit with some cookies involved, Sharon used her personality to convince John to take a job helping Nate at the JT Ranch. Sharon "loaned" Nancy's buggy to John and a horse to travel to the ranch. She explained that this would allow him to help Nate for a longer period. At first, John thought he was doing the Johnsons a big favor. He started out working two days a week at the JT Ranch. Nate thanked him often for his help, and Sharon finished off each day with dinner for the Jacobs, along with her kind words for John's help.

As time passed, John started working more days. The JT needed his help, and he could use the work. It didn't take long for Sharon to convince Mr. Jacobs to come early on the days he worked at the ranch. She mentioned that Nate and she fixed breakfast every morning. It wouldn't be much harder to prepare a little more. Sharon also volunteered to help get Elizabeth ready for school. After stating that he wanted the breakfast costs to come out of his pay, Mr. Jacobs agreed. The girls loved coming over.

On school days, Sharon would help Elizabeth get ready while Ruthie put on her "work clothes". Mrs. Johnson and Ruthie would take Lizzie to school and pick her up. Sharon taught Ruthie many things as they did chores. Ruthie never liked taking a nap before, but she always took one for Sharon. Nate loved watching the two as they went about the day. He especially liked it when they held hands. Sharon always spent some time with Lizzie after school. She would ask about the school day and help with any homework. Nate would help with Ruthie. Ruthie enjoyed this time, as did Nate. Sharon babysat both girls on Saturdays. She mentored the girls on many subjects. Ruthie and Lizzie were becoming very attached to the Johnsons. WHO WOULD NOT.

The Moore family came to town about five weeks after Nate and Sharon's wedding. Thomas spotted them coming into town on a Monday morning. They had a fully packed Calistoga wagon. They looked tired and, obviously, had been on the road for some time. Thomas walked over and introduced himself. He smiled and asked if he could be of any assistance. The husband introduced himself and everybody in the family. He explained they had been on the Fort Smith-Santa Fe Trail, but the family had been delayed in Fort Smith while Wyatt recovered from an illness. It was too late to travel on to Santa Fe, so they were looking for a place to winter down and find work.

Thomas smiled again and said, "Michelle, Tom, Wyatt, and Mike, It is very nice to make your acquaintance. I think I might be of some assistance. My buggy is just across the street. Follow me for about a mile; we'll see if the couple you'll meet can help you with a few things."

Nate and Sharon were working in the garden getting everything ready for the canning to begin. Nate was excited because his boss in this entire process just happened to be his amazing and talented wife. He never got tired of working together with Sharon. They spotted Thomas a ways off, wondering why he was coming out to the ranch as he had said he would be busy all day in town. He wasn't expected until tomorrow afternoon. As he arrived, they spotted the covered wagon coming down the road. Thomas simply said as he exited the buggy, "We need to help these folks."

After introductions, Tom Moore explained everything to the Johnsons, including some of the family's skills. Michelle was willing to do most work that women normally do, and she was accomplished at sewing. Tom mentioned that he was a jack-of-all-trades. He would take any type of work. The boys were big enough to assist on any physical work along with any chores around the ranch. He explained that Wyatt will need some more time to get his strength back, but he can still be of assistance. Mr. Moore seemed like a good man judging from his demeanor and mannerisms. This was a nice family.

Sharon took charge after Nate squeezed her hand three times. She told the Moores, "You would be doing us a huge favor if you would occupy a little house about a half mile away. It has been empty for some time. We didn't know what to do with it; now we do. It is small, but maybe we could help you build a small addition. We were actually going over today to harvest the garden. We can do that now if my wonderful husband hitches up the wagon." Sharon was so personable; her smiles and style made the Moores feel welcomed. Thomas and Nate both loved it. She had truly blossomed as a person, especially with children.

The group headed over to Sharon's old place. Michelle, Nate, and Sharon went to the garden as Thomas showed the people around the ranch. This was Sharon's plan that she had quickly mentioned to her people while the Moores were heading back to their wagon. She wanted to get the work done in the garden and leave the family alone to settle into their new home. They might appreciate some privacy. Sharon told Michelle to come back to the JT Ranch around 1 p.m. for lunch. They would talk about work at that time. Sharon had a very good feeling about Michelle.

Thomas left before lunch; he had work back in town. Thomas mentioned that he would pay the Moores for any work that the JT Ranch couldn't recoup. It was the least he could do since he was the one to bring this family to Nate and Sharon. Thomas wanted Nate and Sharon to orchestrate a design that enabled them to feel good about helping. This was their second time doing a significant good deed, but he didn't want it to be too costly. He thanked them for helping. The kind vet said he had a good feeling about a family; everything is going to be great. Nate and Sharon fixed a simple lunch right after Thomas left. They discussed the work the Moores might do as they put lunch together.

The Moore family had cleaned up and changed into some nice clothes. The Johnsons noticed. They both thought it was respectful, a nice gesture but didn't say anything. Instead, they focused on the boys. Sharon stated that it must be nice to have two strong boys to help with chores. Both parents pointed out how helpful the twins were. Sharon asked the boys directly about school. Mrs. Johnson had, of course, been the one to welcome them back. Nate was smiling and pleasant, but he knew his wife had the charisma and pretty smile to make everybody feel welcome at the ranch.

Nate and Sharon explained some of the jobs they needed to be performed as the group walked around the ranch. The ranch owners found out that the twins were very good with horses. They could chop wood and fall a tree. Michelle had taught them quite a lot about gardens. Tom explained that the boys had finished their schooling back in May. Since that time until they moved in the first part of August, the boys have been learning different jobs around the farm. They are good workers. They will even milk the goats and make you some cheese.

Michelle stated that she didn't have many skills besides sewing. Sharon jumped in with a big smile, along with the words that she would make Michelle the head of the sewing department since nobody else here can sew. Nate mentioned how he and Sharon struggle to sew something that he has torn. He told Michelle, "You have a very valuable skill to share. Please thank your nimble fingers." He smiled, as did Sharon. Sharon could tell that Michelle appreciated the nice comments.

Tom told Nate that he worked at a lumber mill when he was young. He was anxious to help Nate cut that fine looking wood lying next to the mill. He could do some carpenter work and harvest wood. He mentioned, "I've made charcoal many times. I'd be happy to help you make some more as I see your supply is running low." He added that he had never seen such great equipment on one ranch. This place is amazing.

Sharon explained to the Moores that the ranch was a wedding gift from Thomas. She figured that they would find out soon enough.

She felt that she could add a different perspective to the story than the one they might get in town. Many people had been very happy for the newlyweds in regards to them receiving such a gift, but there were some who were still quite jealous. Sharon needed the Moores to know who Dr. Thomas Smith was. It would be nice if they knew his plans for the JT Ranch.

All four Moores were shocked at such a humongous and expensive gift. Sharon told them that Nate and Thomas are like a father and son; they couldn't be any closer. Thomas has known Nate pretty much his whole life. He is a veterinarian, but, more importantly, he is a very intelligent man with the kindest heart. He and his late wife, Marjorie, have mentored Nate since he was a young boy. They taught Nate so much about so many topics. Marjorie was the lead mentor. Nate says she was simply unbelievable. The Smiths always believed that every day was a chance to do good deeds and be a positive influence. The Moores are now a recipient of that philosophy.

The man who owned this ranch before us was evil. He did much harm to this town. There's no sense in getting into the details. Sharon told the Moores, "You'll find out as you visit with people in town. Dr. Smith and his good friend, Dan Perkins, are changing this town in a very positive way. Thomas felt that we could do good things with this ranch. He wanted us to continue the Smiths' legacy. We intend to do so. It gives us great joy to be like the Smiths. You will find that there is no better man alive than Dr. Thomas Smith. We will try to follow in his footsteps."

Nate stated that he and Sharon didn't know much about wages. Tom asked about the soldiers on the weekends. Nate explained, "We don't pay them anything. My beautiful and intelligent wife came up with a plan that benefits everyone. That's what she does with most people she meets. Anyway, we give the army one of our prized cows every occasionally in place of wages for the part time wranglers. The soldiers love the work, the army loves the beef, and we love the help. This ranch has great cattle, the best in the entire area. Sharon is in charge of the cattle operation here at the JT. She is a great cowboy and knows so much. This is why Michelle will be invaluable.

Michelle's work will let Sharon visit her 'four legged friends' while riding Rusty, her second best friend."

Michelle, once again, appreciated the comments. Thomas, Nate, and Sharon had rescued a family of strangers in need. They could have put some demands on the newcomers that would have had to be met, or, if not, they would have been sent packing. Surely the Johnsons knew that the Moores were getting desperate for a place to stay. Michelle was so appreciative. These kind people had opened up their homes and hearts to total strangers. She had been very concerned about Wyatt with winter on the way and no place to stay. Now they had a small house to keep him warm and well fed until he fully recovers. She was so happy; she really liked Nate and Sharon.

After a pleasant lunch and a nice visit, it was decided that the Moores would start work tomorrow. Nate and Tom would fire up the lumber mill. Michelle would help Sharon with the canning. The boys would tend to the animals, chop some wood, and maybe make some cheese. Nate and Tom started loading up the wagon with some feed for the horses, a two-man saw, a very sharp ax, and a small supply of kindling and firewood. The guest was very appreciative. He stated that he would pay the Johnsons back as soon as possible. Nate thanked him for the offer, but he explained, "Everything we're giving you was left by Nancy, the owner of the ranch before us. She wanted us to give it away." As the men were loading the wagon, the boys checked out all the animals again. They were very impressed with all the horses the Johnsons owned.

After several minutes, the whole group gathered at the wagon. Sharon provided enough canned goods for dinner along with eggs and bacon for tomorrow morning. She also provided the biscuits she had made for her and Nate's dinner and breakfast. There was also a jar of her famous jam. Just before the family left, Nate explained to them that he sometimes calls his wife a cowboy instead of a cowgirl. It is meant as the best compliment possible because her skills are better than most men are. She is extremely talented and calling her, a cowgirl doesn't seem to convey that. He further explained that he loves Sharon's many talents and she loves mine. His last words to the

Moores as they mounted the wagon were, "Sharon and I are very glad you are here. You will be a huge help to us."

Wyatt and Mike tended to the horses when they arrived "home" while Tom and Michelle finished moving in. Michelle told her husband that she just had to ask Sharon who her best friend was while Sharon was getting all the food together. Michelle explained that she already knew the answer but wanted to hear Sharon's response. Michelle informed her husband that the female cowboy's best friend is Nate. It seems that these newlyweds really enjoy working together, spending time together, and talking together. Michelle mentioned this because she and her husband had not done those things very often lately. Tom responded, "I have been under so much stress lately. I will make an effort to do better. I really like being settled. We were very lucky to find work and this place."

Nate and Sharon loved their afternoon together; being alone allowed them to focus on the canning process and enjoy the activity together. Sharon was so impressed with Nate's focus and his ability with his hands. He was so strong, yet he had fine skills with his hands. He caught on quickly and really seemed to enjoy the work. Nate thoroughly enjoyed the activity with Sharon. The way she gave directions and suggestions reminded him of Marjorie doing the same thing in the garden when he was young. The smiles, the mannerisms, and the touches were very much alike. The more she praised his work, the more he complimented her techniques and knowledge. The biggest difference between working with T compared to M was the fact that Nate loved the benefits of working with Sharon. There were many hugs and kisses.

After dinner was completed, the couple decided to write a couple of letters – Nate to his father and Sharon to Mary. Nate's letter was straight forward – information about the ranch and their new guests. He injected some humor along with the request to receive a letter from the whole family. Each person could write a short note on what they were doing. Nate stated that he would really like that.

Sharon's letter was going to take more time. She knew that Nate's would be done in thirty minutes. Her letter was personable and emotional; it would take quite a bit longer. It took her three days to finish the letter. There were minutes that went by when she wrote nothing. A couple of times she started over, but she finally was satisfied with what she had written. She started out by explaining why she had chosen to call Mary – M2. "That name even means something special to me; I can only imagine what it means to you. I know that it is impossible to reach the love and admiration that M and M2 had together, but I want you to know that I have started to develop those two emotions for you. My father damaged my mother. She wasn't able to love me as if I know she wanted to. You have been so kind and loving to me in the short time that we have been connected. Thank you"

Sharon talked about the new family that just arrived. "Thomas had seen them in town and knew they needed help. It looks like they will be able to spend the winter helping around the ranch. They are staying at my old place. It is rather nice because we need the help, and they need the jobs. The Moores have twin boys about thirteen who seem to have some skills to help with the work."

Sharon invited the Johnsons out for a visit after the spring rains. She wanted M2 to tell her more stories about Marjorie. Sharon explained, "I use the lessons that Nate has taught me in my dealings with others. These powerful things were taught to him by you and M." The newlywed added, "The more that I can learn from you and Nate, the more good deeds I can perform. I just want to thank you for everything you have done for me. M has left a legacy that may never be matched. You were her best friend and have done similar things. It will be hard to measure up to what you two have accomplished, but with Nate's help I hope to do half as well as you two have."

Nate and Tom went to work immediately at the mill as soon as Tom arrived. Nate knew some things about the steam engine. He listened to his "expert's" instructions. The fire was built, the pressure rose to the correct temperature, and the saw was started. Everything was running smoothly. Tom explained Nate's job to him. Mr. Moore positioned and measured the piece of wood to be cut. Things were all set; Nate wanted to review his job again with Tom again just to make sure. Nate remembered everything; they were all set to cut. They cut the first log into ten one inch pieces of lumber and then stopped the operation for a minute to check out their work.

Tom explained to Nate that you always look at the first cuts to see how the saw is operating. Mr. Moore said that sometimes the sound of the saw tells you how things are going. He said that this mill is in excellent condition, and this wood is high quality. He also mentioned that at his old job they usually made standard planks from average wood. We always kept wood like this for special orders. This wood would be expensive. It would be used to make furniture. Nate told Tom that he would use this wood to make birdhouses and possibly some small furniture with Thomas' help. The kind old vet is quite good with wood. Nate said that there was a tree nearby that he wanted to cut down. It is a pine tree. Would that be good?

Tom replied, "Yes, let's go bring it down."

The men talked about pay as they worked. Nate told Tom that he didn't know how busy the mill would be for the near future. People don't normally build in the winter. We only have two months of halfway decent weather left. Let us cut enough wood to fill the wagon. We will take it to the next town market and see how it goes. Tom asked what the town market was. Nate explained everything. The newcomer's only response was that this Dr. Smith seems like quite a person.

Nate simply said, "He is a great man with many talents."

Nate asked Tom if it seemed fair that the people working the mill split sixty percent of the sales with the other forty going to the ranch for upkeep and profit. He also mentioned that Thomas knows the price of lumber. He stated, "Sharon and I definitely want to be fair to our neighbors. Our prices will generally be on the low side." He told his hired hand that he could advertise at the town market to sell firewood. There is always a need for wood, especially with winter coming. People prefer dried wood. Some trees on the property are dying. You and the boys can have those for a small fee determined by you. You can also use Thomas' wagon and our horses free. Nate thought it was important not to give too many things to the Moores. Men generally don't like that. He knew Mr. Moore would pay something for the use of the wagon and be fair in paying for the trees.

Tom could not believe how quick and hard Nate could work. He had always fancied himself as a very good worker, strong with good endurance, but he couldn't keep up with Nate. He asked for a break several times when they were operating the two-man saw. Mr. Moore was starting to be impressed with this young man. He was definitely skilled with wood and iron. He was starting to get curious about a man who seemed to treat his wife as an equal. Tom was definitely not raised that way in the rural parts of Tennessee. It was something that he would consider. Mr. Moore was, very definitely, thankful for the house and the work. He would, in the end, learn so much from the three people who had befriended him and his family. After the one and a half years while they lived at Sharon's old place and worked at the JT Ranch, all the Moores left for California thankful for all the things that had transpired.

Sharon and Michelle had a very productive day canning; they worked well together. Both were very experienced, as they each had been canning for most of their lives. They laughed and made jokes about their mistakes of the past. With all the laughs and smiles, the two women became instant friends. Sharon found out that Michelle was two years older than she was. Michelle found out that Sharon had been married before. Michelle, like Sharon in her first marriage, hadn't really had any friends back in Tennessee. She really appreciated having someone to share chores with; she loved the conversation.

When the Moores left for California, Michelle was so saddened to leave. She would miss her best friend that made everybody she met, happier and better off. Mrs. Moore really appreciated the changes in her husband. He was kinder, treated her more as an equal, listened to her opinions, and was more affectionate. Nate and Sharon were responsible for this. Michelle's life was so much better. Mrs. Moore knew the family plan was to buy land in California. Tom wanted to develop something special for the boys to have one day. Michelle did not want to leave, but the family plan made sense. The move had to happen.

During the entire time Michelle was there at the JT Ranch, Sharon was able to manage the cattle with a more hands on approach. Some days Thomas rode out with her. She and Thomas always thought that the hired hands had "helped" themselves to a number of the herd, not many, but enough to build a small nest egg. This stopped with Thomas and Sharon monitoring all cattle activities. The number of cattle grew to about 250; the income also grew. Nate couldn't believe how lucrative the cattle business was.

The JT Ranch was highly profitable; money was also coming in from Nate's blacksmith work, John and Tom's lumber and firewood sales, Mike and Wyatt's sales, and revenue from the town market. Nate had talked to Sharon many times about buying some nice things for herself. She explained to Nate that she remembered Marjorie's lesson about money. She knew that the Johnson's were not rich yet, but she would never want to appear in public dressed up to demonstrate wealth. She loved the clothes that Michelle was making for her. They were very well made, original, and quite colorful, which Sharon really enjoyed. Michelle loved the compliments from the Johnsons and Dr. Smith. Tom also thanked her for all the money she was bringing in. She had actually sold a number of different types of clothing to many women in town.

Many times when discussing ranch business, Sharon would put her arms around Nate, kiss him on the cheek, and ask him who his favorite cowboy was. Nate always responded in the perfect fashion. She loved it when every occasionally in public, he would call her the best cowboy he ever knew. Sharon could definitely ride with the best of them and rope like a champion.

Sharon taught Wyatt and Mike how to ride and rope. She thought it was a skill they might use in California. John Jacobs taught the boys how to dress out a cow. It took several lessons, but, in the end, the boys could handle the chore by themselves. Nate always paid them, explaining that they were doing men's work and should be paid like men. Thank you Jack Brown. In time, the two boys were also making the charcoal for the ranch and the town. There was no doubt that the Moores were thriving at the JT Ranch. There were many meals shared with the Moores, Johnsons, and Dr. Smith. Nate could not help thinking that these meals reminded him of the countless meals between the Smiths and his family when he was younger. Thomas and Sharon always led the conversation at the meals, sharing their constant smiles and compliments.

Occasionally, the Jacobs would share a meal with the group. John was still a quiet man, but Nate observed that he seemed to enjoy the company. He did laugh and smile often at the table. Wyatt and Mike were very kind to Elizabeth and Ruthie. They played with the girls before and after dinner. The girls loved it, as did the boys. Their favorite toy was Winny.

Shortly after returning from the wedding, the Johnsons noticed Bee, Sharon's mare that she used to pull the buggy, was pregnant. Sharon then remembered that one soldier on "babysitting duty" had said that Bee was friendly with one of the army horses. Winny appeared on the scene eleven months later. She was adorable. Sharon saw Nate's vet skills firsthand as he watched over Bee the entire time. Thomas observed but wanted Nate to be in charge. Nate loved showing his wife his skills. Sharon loved learning new things about horses. It was another thing they enjoyed doing together. In the years to come, they would deliver over two dozen foals.

After several meals, John joined the men on the porch where they discussed work and town business as they watched the children play. He learned to share more of his thoughts with these new friends. He really enjoyed listening to Thomas' words about everything. He had become a big fan of this amazing man. The retired vet never bragged about anything and John never heard a negative word spoken from Thomas. He would remember these things.

Sharon and Michelle really enjoyed the atmosphere of these occasions. Everyone was happy with the friendly interaction. The two women enjoyed cooking and cleaning up together. Of course, they had to shoo Nate and Thomas out of the kitchen in the beginning, but the two men grew to enjoy Tom and John's company. This allowed the two women friends to enjoy their "women's" talk. Nate and Thomas realized that Sharon and Michelle's talks when alone were similar to the ones M and M2 had.

Sharon occasionally took Nate out to a faraway pasture to shoot rifles and pistols. Thomas declined the invitation because he wanted Sharon to teach Nate how to improve his skills. It would give her great pleasure. He was right. On one particular shoot, Nate explained to Sharon that their private time, working together, either shooting, or whatever comes up, rejuvenates his happiness for the world. He said, "I don't completely understand it, but my dearest wife makes me so happy. You completely fill me up with joy, and it spills out to others as I see them. You make me a better man." The shooting stopped for a short time.

One Sunday after church, Sharon invited the Moores to go on a picnic. She mentioned that it is also a place where Nate and she do some practice shooting. Wyatt and Mike were so excited that Tom agreed to go. Sharon noted that Michelle hadn't been asked. Michelle did mention in one of her talks with Sharon that her husband was changing. It was going to be a work in progress. They were now holding hands on some occasions and were talking more than they had ever done before. This is all because of the Johnsons.

Tom had never seen Sharon do any cowboy work, but he did a short time later. Mrs. Johnson, on the ride out to the picnic, was wearing a colorful and charming cowgirl outfit made by Michelle. Nate loved the design and colors. He had thanked Michelle several times when she first made it. As the group neared the pasture they were going to use, a stray calf went ambling right across everyone's view. In a few seconds, Sharon's rope was out, and she rode hard to intercept the "little dogie". In under ten seconds, she had the calf roped and tied off. Nate was following the action close behind. He put the calf in front of his saddle and delivered the little person back to his mother.

Nate and Sharon were still laughing about it as the group reached their picnic area.

Lunch was very enjoyable. This area of the ranch was stunning. The Moores had never been out this far and were very impressed. Sharon had made a new flavor of jam, and the whole crew loved it. Nate said it was the best jam he'd ever had. Tom agreed 100%. He was becoming a big fan of Sharon's cooking, not to mention her tasty jams. He now understood what Nate had said about Sharon being the best cowboy he'd ever seen. SHE WAS VERY GOOD!

The shooting practice started after lunch. Tom had brought out two rifles that were his dad's. They were good, but didn't compare to the ones Thomas had given to the

Johnsons. Mr. Moore only shot his rifle explaining that he needed to be proficient with it as it is the one he uses. Sharon agreed with his thoughts completely. He did say it was okay for the boys to shoot the Johnsons' rifles. Nate and the boys had a friendly competition. Nate was really getting good at hitting some small targets. Sharon knew he would let the boys win, even though he was a better shot. He did. That was only a small part of why she loved him so much, always putting others' feelings before his own.

As the shooting wound down for the day, Tom asked if Sharon was going to shoot. She explained that sometimes she does; other times she just likes to watch. She told the boys that they were good shots. Sharon smiled as she said their performance was excellent. Mr. Moore asked Sharon if she would please shoot. Tom asked for just two shots. The boys would love it. Sharon was quite surprised that Tom asked her to shoot with the word please included in the request. She agreed, and Nate set up the targets. The first one was a small pinecone next to the cans the men were shooting. It was small compared to the cans. Nate then set up a pinecone on a nearby rock. Sharon hit the distant pinecone on the first shot, stood up, quickly drew her pistol from its holster, and hit the nearby pinecone. The boys went crazy. Michelle was clapping with the biggest smile on her face.

Mr. Moore was shaking his head and said, "I have never seen such fine shooting in my entire life. You are amazingly talented."

Sharon nodded her head and touched her cowboy hat. She only shot to let Tom know that women have skills; all women skills need to be appreciated. Mrs. Johnson knew of

Michelle's skills. She was hoping that Tom would start to appreciate his wife's skills also.

Michelle was a wonderful cook, and her sewing skills were extraordinary. She taught Sharon how to sew along with some of the finer points of raising boys. Sharon really appreciated the sewing lessons; they would come in handy. She found the lessons about boys very interesting. Michelle was kind but firm with the boys. She explained things thoroughly and always asked the boys if they understood. She smiled often when talking to her sons. Sharon liked that. She wasn't sure she'd ever mentor boys, but you never know.

Nate and Sharon grew much attached to Elizabeth and Ruthie, especially Sharon. She grew to become their surrogate mother. John grew to appreciate the help, as he knew he couldn't handle the job. Some things just needed a woman's skills and knowledge. Mrs. Johnson really missed Ruthie when she started school. Luckily, Nate was there with all the right things to make the transition less painful. Once again, Sharon has to spend more time during the day with Nate. That would fix anything.

One more thing that Sharon and Nate really did like was Thomas' new friend, Delores Martin; her friends call her Dee. She became instant friends with Sharon and Nate. They were very happy for Dee and Thomas. The new couple seemed to enjoy walks after dinner and buggy rides out to the country. They smiled and laughed when they were together. The relationship gave the kind vet something to do in the evenings; Dee was great company. Thomas also wanted some distance from the couple that he enjoyed so much. He loved them dearly, but they needed their space to grow into the couple that would benefit this town in so many ways.

The Johnsons were off to a great start. The people in town knew of the great things the JT Ranch was providing to the Jacobs and Moores. The ranch provided the jobs, but it was the kindness towards strangers that really impressed everyone. People had seen Nate and Sharon interact with the four children. It was touching to see how much the two adults valued the children. The three families had become very friendly; everybody was enjoying, supporting, and encouraging each other. It was a pleasure to see. This was exactly what Thomas wanted to see happen. The JT Ranch was allowing Nate and Sharon to do good deeds and be a positive influence.

Chapter 15

A Big Visit

The Johnson clan came to visit during the first summer after Nate and Sharon's wedding. They were so impressed with the house. M2 said that she might never leave. Jeremy asked if he could work at the mill for a day. He had always wanted to make finished wood for construction. Doris and Andy wanted to ride horses. On the second day of their visit, Sharon and Thomas took Andy and Doris riding. They rode out to the property line where they were thrilled to see the wild horses. Both kids couldn't believe how big the ranch was. It was a very memorable ride. As it turned out, John and Tom were scheduled to take down a couple of trees. This allowed Nate and his father to work the mill. Jeremy really enjoyed learning all about the workings of this wood-producing enterprise. Nate was thrilled to actually teach his father something.

After leaving his father later that day to work on a furniture project, the young co-owner of the ranch went to the kitchen where he helped his mother prepare dinner. Several months later, Mary informed Mabel that fixing dinner with Nate that afternoon was one of the highlights of her life. Her son reminded her so much of Thomas and Marjorie. Nate was a joy to be around. He made his mother smile and laugh all the while they were preparing dinner. M2 didn't understand it at first, but she figured that Sharon was the primary factor in Nate's personality. Mary would have to tell Sharon again why she was the reason for this.

After dinner, Doris and Andy wanted to do the dishes. Nate and Jeremy went back to work on the furniture project. Jeremy had really enjoyed the work in the afternoon and wanted to get back to it. Nate was more than happy to join him. He loved it when the both of them worked together on projects. Nate liked watching his father do intricate woodwork. He learned so much. As the men left, Mary asked Sharon, "Would you please walk with me, so I can see your beautiful ranch."

M2 mentioned on the walk how much she enjoyed making dinner with her son. She explained to Sharon, "Nate was charming in so many ways. He was also much more talented in the kitchen than I remember, but you already knew that." I would like to focus on why he was so personable. There is a rather simple answer as to why my darling son has become so friendly. You have helped make him charming and personable because you have filled him with so much love and happiness. Psalm 23 mentions "My cup runneth over". "Nate is like that cup. Happiness pours out of him because he has so much inside him. I know I've said things like this in the past, but I need to tell you many times how thankful I am for you."

Sharon explained that from the moment she met Thomas she started to learn from him. It had nothing to do with book stuff. It was all about feelings and interactions with people. She mentioned that she had not really ever had any friends before, but she viewed Thomas as a friend right after they met. She had never experienced anything like it before in her life. She laughed and smiled in Thomas' company so much. She really started to enjoy the friendship. She started to look to him as the father figure she never had. She enjoyed his personable touches to her arm or shoulder as he gave her compliments. "I grew to want to hug him when we met. I never hugged my dad or mother, but I really wanted to hug this wonderful man. Thomas always extended his hand when we met. He would hold my hand for a short time as we said our hellos. I always figured that he didn't want to cross any lines. I looked forward to visiting with Thomas so much that I would stop by his place."

Mary was starting to derive a conclusion. She wondered if Thomas knew this woman was the perfect fit for Nate. Did he have a premonition of what was going to happen to Sharon's husband? Was he teaching Sharon things from Marjorie that he knew Nate would appreciate and grow to love? M2 knew that M was guiding Thomas on many topics during their years of mentoring Nate. Thomas was an excellent teacher. He was very capable of delivering the perfect lesson, and Mary knew that Marjorie possessed an uncanny ability as to when and how to teach Nate. When Mary's son was ready for more advanced lessons that required higher levels of emotional and social development, M would provide all the aspects needed to guarantee

Nate's success. Thomas was an invaluable aide who knew the entire plan. Marjorie realized that Nate needed a male role model to emulate.

Thomas knew how to "read" people very quickly. Did he realize that Sharon was damaged? She was lacking love and support, two of the most basic needs of life, according to Marjorie. Could Thomas use the things Marjorie taught him to open up Sharon's heart and mind to love, kindness, and support? The kind vet knew that Nate would enjoy Sharon's love for horses, her ability to do fine work, and that marvelous smile she was exhibiting more and more often during her visits with him. Nate was a very kind man who knew how to compliment and support others. Sharon would quickly grow to love Nate's words. Was Marjorie's right hand man attempting to get these two talented people together?

Mary knew that Nate was interested in finding someone to start a relationship with. Pulling him from school at eleven prevented him from some of the social interactions where he might have met someone, but she knew he was not ready for a girlfriend until Marjorie had worked her "magic". When Nate was twenty-one, he told his mother one day that he wanted to experience the love of a spouse. There was no doubt that if Mary knew this fact, M and Thomas also knew.

The kind old doctor knew that there would be an explosion of love and affection once Nate and Sharon were put together. Mary also knew that Thomas was a person who often gave a friendly hug to the women he knew, never too much, but perfectly appropriate. She would ask Sharon one question that would explain just about everything. Mary suspected that, once again, there was a distinct possibility that divine intervention may have been involved in putting these two people together. Thomas had been confident that Marjorie had been at the wedding.

As the two women neared the house after their walk, Mary asked, "Sharon, Has anybody touched your heart in the last five years?"

Sharon quickly answered, "My Nate. It was a hug and a kiss on the cheek that I will never forget. He held me tight for quite some time and then whispered 'I've got you'. I had never been hugged like that before; his arms held me tight, but his hands were gentle. His voice was kind and caring."

Mary smiled as they reached the house. She took Sharon's hand and squeezed it for about two seconds. Maybe she should write Thomas a thank you letter. When the kind vet left Sharon's place on that dreadful day, he knew that Nate would embrace Sharon. It was the correct thing to do. He also knew that the embrace would be magical for both people. IT WAS.

Mary guided Sharon off to the side for a minute where she whispered, "Can I call you G in my letters and when we're having a private conversation?

"Of course you can, M2," said Sharon as she took Mary's hands. "I'd love that." She returned Mary's affectionate hand squeeze to both of her mother-in-law's hands.

When both women entered the house, they were very happy to have such a close relationship. They seemed to really enjoy each other's company. Once inside, Sharon wanted to show Mary the outfits Michelle had made for her. M2 was very impressed; she liked the design and especially loved the color combinations. G said that she was learning to sew. She couldn't wait to make outfits for the girls. Sharon mentioned that she and Nate would love another visit next summer. She apologized for not being able to travel away from the ranch, but they didn't have the help to keep things in working order. Thomas was busy with several things, and, although he would never say no, they just couldn't ask. Mary said that everyone loves coming here. It would be a joy to come next summer. Sharon smiled when M2 said, "We could do some sewing together."

In the morning, the visiting Johnson clan was on hand to meet John, Elizabeth, and Ruthie. John was polite but quickly excused himself as not to keep Tom waiting. Everyone understood. Nate and his father headed for the wood shop. M2 told Sharon that she would handle the dishes with help from Doris. Andy had decided to go with the people to work with wood. He was starting to really enjoy the activity. Sharon took the girls upstairs where she fixed their hair. She had bought them new outfits; they were very excited.

Mary joined them when they came downstairs. The former teacher watched carefully throughout the morning as the three did their chores. The girls listened to Sharon's every word. It did not take much observation skills to realize these two little girls adored Sharon. Early on in the day, Mary couldn't believe what she was witnessing. Sharon was a natural with little ones; she was very much like Marjorie. Her smiles, compliments, and conversation made the girls so happy to help with the chores.

Mary smiled when the three workers got to the garden. Sharon drifted off towards the horses as Elizabeth took charge. Ruthie even called her captain a few times. Mary loved the interaction between the girls. She followed them out to the farm animals where the roles were reversed. Elizabeth was so kind to her little sister. She listened intently; she asked questions if something was not clear. It was cute to watch. Mary was thrilled that her little lesson to teach her children how to work and get along had been passed on to Sharon.

After lunch, Nate insisted that his mother and father go on a buggy ride to view the ranch and the cattle. While on the ride, they were so impressed with everything. They walked around in many places in order to see the beautiful scenery. Mary mentioned now that Doris was leaving for college in a month and Andy getting ready to move on from grade school, it might be time for them to discuss their plans. Jeremy surprised Mary by what he said. She knew he was growing somewhat tired of being a minister. The town was losing population; there was talk of reducing his pay, maybe even ending his job. A minister's job can involve many hours of counseling and comforting. Jeremy had been a splendid minister for over twenty-one years.

Mary listened as her husband said, "I've considered quitting the ministry. I have thoroughly enjoyed it, but, at times, I am growing tired of performing the job. I told myself many years ago that I would quit the ministry if it became a strain. I am almost at that point. Seeing this place makes me want to be here."

Mary told Jeremy that she absolutely loves it here. Let us talk to Nate and Sharon. When they arrived back at the house, Thomas was there. It was a touching reunion. Thomas was extremely happy to see the four visiting Johnsons. Mary was somewhat surprised when this fine man introduced his woman friend, Delores Martin. She knew this friend had to be someone special. He would not bring just anyone to this reunion dinner. Delores said during the introductions that her friends call her Dee. Mary knew immediately one of the main reasons why Thomas liked this woman; her smile was very pleasant. Sharon whispered to Mary as everyone headed towards the house that she would bet anyone a penny that Thomas and Dee are married within a year. Mary smiled and squeezed Sharon's hand.

In the first fifteen minutes of dinner, Thomas talked constantly. He explained things about each person at the table, made jokes, and kept everyone smiling. Mary and Sharon both knew he was excited. Mary whispered to her daughter-in-law that she had been right about these two. Dee and Thomas were very good together.

After everyone had been introduced to Dee, Mary smiled, took Thomas' hand, and said, "You have made us thrilled with your enhanced introductions of the traveling band of Johnsons. Thank you for the kind words. We are so fortunate to have you as a member of the clan. Now you can make your stomach happy as I have an announcement to make. Jeremy and I will be talking to Andy very soon and Nate and Sharon somewhat later about," she paused for longer than necessary, "moving here."

Everyone started talking at once, but Mary and Sharon were honed in on Andy's words and reactions. Sharon knew that the Johnsons would not move at this time without his approval. He was thirteen, had some friends, and was quite settled. The move might come later. Sharon sure hoped the move would happen. Mary was very aware that she had leveraged the situation in front of everybody. It was something she had never done before, but she truly believed that Andy would do so much better here than at home. The smile on

Andy's face, along with the words "I love it", pretty much confirmed the move would happen.

Sharon stood up and spoke with quite a bit of emotion, "This is so much more than wonderful. Nate and I can't wait. Thank you in advance for joining us. We love you; we love that you are moving here. We've been very blessed; now, it's going to be ten times better." IT WAS.

Chapter 16

The Johnson Clan

One day when Nate was about twenty-eight, he was taking a break from work to have some water. He started thinking about all the great things that had transpired since his marriage. So much of it revolved around Sharon. She meant so much too so many people. Mrs. Johnson was the most considerate, kind boss anyone could imagine. She always explained the entire job to her employees. Therefore, there was no misunderstanding. She expected a full day of quality work. She would praise and congratulate every worker on a job well done if it was deserved. She smiled often and seemed to really value each worker. Her workers did not want to disappoint Sharon. Nate loved watching her dealing with people in general. Her words, her smile, and her positive concern for others made her very popular. She was very special.

Sharon had been a splendid teacher to the Moores. She taught Mike and Wyatt a number of things and always supported their work habits with wonderful compliments. They really liked Sharon's smile, along with the fact that Mrs. Johnson knew so much about so many things. The twins were indeed highly impressed with the best cowboy they had ever seen, even though the cowboy was a woman.

Tom and Michelle had a completely different relationship after spending about one and a half years at the JT Ranch. Michelle thanked Sharon several times, for what she did. Tom learned to appreciate his wife's skills. They both truly valued what Sharon taught them. Nate and Sharon really liked the sign the Moore family made. Tom hung it at the lumber mill after all four finished the carving. At the top, Tom put, in big letters, the words "To Nate and Sharon" and right below, the message "Words cannot describe our thanks for your kindness and friendship". Each other family member carved a short message and, right below, their first name. Each person's lettering was quite different by design. Nate knew the family had spent many hours making the sign. Nate and Sharon loved the sign. Some days after dinner, they would walk out to the mill to see the sign. It brought such joy. Thomas' eyes watered the first time he saw it. He was so proud.

Nate loved what Sharon did for the entire Moore family. Sharon had helped them in so many ways. Nate sat there in awe of his wife. He always thought it was an equal to M; she may have done even better with the Moores than Marjorie could have done. He did not think that was possible; that is why he sat there, utterly amazed.

Several years ago when Sharon was talking to John one day, she happened to say the words "my girls". She quickly apologized. John responded, "There is no need to apologize. They are your girls. They have learned so much from you; they talk about you constantly. I was jealous for a short time, but I then realized that you were and continue to be a supreme benefit to my daughters. I will always be their dad and will try to provide whatever I can to further their growth, but you are the girls' mentor, their support and comfort, and are guiding them with so much love. You are simply amazing. The girls view you as their stepmom. The Jacobs family loves what you do, and I might add that Nate is the greatest uncle in the world. The girls love him too."

The young strong blacksmith liked reminiscing about those words from John. After Sharon shared with Nate John's opinion about the greatest uncle in the world, she kissed him. Wow, Nate thought; he wondered if life could ever get any better than he felt at that particular moment. Again, without Sharon by his side, he wouldn't have a great feeling of emotion. Sharon had seen a need, stepped in to help, and brought Nate along to help. WONDERFUL!

As Nate walked over to check on the horses, he continued thinking about his wife. She spoke often at town meetings held in the square. Sometimes she would talk with Thomas beforehand about what words to use; she always talked with Nate. Somehow, she would blend all the thoughts into a wonderful speech. Thomas said that it is a gift from God. It is a blend of facts, logic, morality, and just the right amount of emotion. Sharon added many smiles and some humor into her speeches. The kind old vet stated that Marjorie had the same skills.

Nate especially liked her speech about children. She started out talking about what great products most of the people in town produce. She did not mention names but explained what great benefits the town enjoys because of its citizens' hard work. She thanked everyone, and then she smiled, paused, and then dropped a statement that surprised everyone except Nate and Thomas, who were smiling. She added, "There is one product that some of you produce that stands far and above anything else we make. CHILDREN they are the future; every one of them needs to be cherished. I am not just talking to the parents. We all can support and encourage good things from our children. I did not misspeak when I said our children. I truly do not want to diminish what parents do. Parents will always do most of the work to raise their offspring, but, every once in a while, we can all assist. It is amazing what a few kind words can do; we all should be able to do that. Please think about what we, as a large supportive group of adults, can accomplish. This town will improve and continue to grow strong because we will have raised such skillful and kind young people. Please help support our children."

The speech was well received by the people of the town. In the next year, Sharon led the group of women who improved the town store and food bank. They added a bulletin board that listed many things available: from part time jobs, pets for adoption, tutoring, farm equipment, to farm animals. The bulletin board was very popular. Some men built some furniture for the store to display; it was free for the asking. There were more used items, some free and others for a greatly reduced price. It was primarily used clothing no longer needed by a particular family. Sharon's goal was that no child should have to be cold in the winter. The store also had some new clothes that were made by the women of the town with fabric provided by the town council members. No one knew it was Nate and Sharon donating the material. Sometimes Sharon would tell some women shoppers to take what they needed. She would pay, and they could do her some favors during the summer months as a payment. This was very popular with some of the women. They loved Sharon for it. SO DID NATE.

Some men in town delivered enough firewood to keep the classrooms warm during the cold months. Two men who lived in town warmed up the rooms every day for the students and teachers. This was very much appreciated by all the teachers who had sometimes seen shivering students sitting in their classes. The teachers, Sharon, and Thomas thanked the men several times for their help. Thomas and Nate knew that these men were setting a new tone for all the males in town; everyone can help in one way or another. Once again, it was Sharon leading the way in helping the children. She was so kind and supportive.

Sharon designed a plan where several people in town prepared a small snack for the children at school every day at 10 a.m. It was explained to the children that they should partake of the snack, unless there was a problem. Appreciate what someone has done for you. Always thank the people who provided the snack. Once a month, many of the children wrote letters to the town council thanking them for sponsoring the snack. The council always shared the letters with the town. The teachers had originally approached Sharon about many of the students having growling stomachs right after recess. Sharon took charge immediately. Mrs. Johnson always wanted to support and encourage children in any way she could. She took note of the ones who might be experiencing the same upbringing as she had endured, but she never mentioned names. Sharon never wanted to embarrass anybody. It would break her heart.

Sharon was constantly praising the work of the town in helping others. One day when she was talking to a group of women in the town square, she used the words "It's a joy to live in a place when the people are so kind. It just warms my heart to be here in such a fine and caring town." Thomas heard the words as he was standing behind Dee, who was part of the group. He quickly turned and walked away from the gathering. He was struck with some powerful emotion. He had heard those exact words from Marjorie about twenty years ago. He smiled as he reminisced about these touching words.

Nate and Sharon shared everything. At night each day, they held hands and talked about their day. One night Sharon thanked Nate for building a couple of shelving units for the town store. She said that they were well done; several women had said so. Nate liked helping to set the tone for the men of the town. Her words made him want to do everything for her. Nate relished his words and work in supporting his wife. It gave him great joy to make her happy. She was doing so much. Another night she explained that several families who the town had helped in earlier times were now contributing items to the food bank and town store. Nate couldn't talk for a few seconds. He simply took Sharon in his arms and held her for some time.

He remembered his exact words as he continued to hold her, "My lovely wife, you are doing such amazing things for so many. You have taught people to give, and that is a wonderful gift to them. People are smiling and laughing, enjoying each other's company. You are helping to make that happen. You do such fantastic things. I couldn't possibly love you anymore; you make me the happiest man on earth."

As Nate was finishing with the horses, he was thinking about how proud he was of his wife. He was also thinking about something she had said a couple of years ago. One night as they were holding hands and talking, Sharon mentioned that her last teacher in school told her that she was the smartest kid he had ever seen. Nate quickly smiled and said that he had always wanted to kiss the smartest kid in class. He did. He explained, "I already knew you were very bright. Every time you enter a room it lights up; now that's bright." She kissed him, and then told him to never tell anyone. Nate held her tighter for a moment and said, "They already know, but I promise I won't say anything."

The JT Ranch allowed him and Sharon to do wonderful things. The ranch was quite an asset in a number of ways. All the hired hands made a nice wage; they also made a profit for the ranch. The people of the town benefitted from reasonable prices of beef, lumber, and iron works. Nate knew Thomas was so proud of what the ranch allowed the Johnsons to do. The old vet knew the Johnsons were quietly helping the town. Sharon told Nate one night, "I like thinking about our good deeds. It gives me great pleasure." Nate quickly gave his wife a big hug and kiss. He loved those words "our good deeds".

Sharon was riding in from a visit with the cattle. The herd was doing well. They were well taken care of because Thomas and Sharon each went out separately at least twice a week. Dan sometimes accompanied the vet; they both enjoyed the excursion. Sharon had moved ten head back to her old place. Twice a week she and Nate cruised over to check out Nate's herd. Sharon named the herd this because her husband was completely in charge. They both truly valued this time together. This was the reason the best cowboy in the family had done it. Every morning and every night Sharon had her Nate time. It never stopped being the best time of the day. Sharon didn't know why she needed to be alone with Nate every day, but she did.

Sharon and Nate's working alone time had dwindled; Many times Mary helped in the garden; this was always pleasant. Sharon was constantly learning things from M2. Mary shared many stories about Marjorie. Although Sharon thoroughly enjoyed the stories, it did cut into her and Nate's special time. Jeremy often groomed the horses right alongside Nate and Sharon. Nate and Sharon enjoyed his father's stories of when he was a child. Nate had never heard them growing up. As great as it was to visit with Jeremy, it did cut into Nate and Sharon's alone time. Having Nate's herd gave the lovable individuals some quality alone time. Nate and Sharon enjoyed the riding, conversation, and herding; they thoroughly enjoyed being a cowboy couple.

One of the many lessons that Nate shared with his wife was that of living a life well lived. It was a long conversation, but one that Sharon really enjoyed. Mrs. Johnson kissed her husband at the end of the lesson, and said that all of his teachings were powerful and very beneficial, but this one stands out as a guiding light on how to live your life. The couple both agreed that helping, supporting, and doing good deeds was the absolute key to a great life. Sharon always kept this particular lesson in her mind.

Several times during their conversations, they mentioned the bully rancher who had hurt so many. Sharon knew some stories that demonstrated his greed and hurtful spirit; she shared these with Nate. The couple talked about what Marjorie had done during her lifetime. Nate shared what he knew about Abigail. Sharon was so impressed with both women. She also mentioned that Nate's mother does good things for people and is a very positive influence. She told her husband that she really loved her mother-in-law. Sharon ended the conversion by telling Nate that she loved his lessons. She was so glad that he was an A+ student. She smiled when she said that, leaned over, and gave him a quick kiss. Sharon thanked him for the grading lesson; she hoped to use it in the near future.

Sharon heard from a number of women in town how muscular and handsome Nate was. The married women were very discreet; the young single women laughed and giggled about Nate. Sharon stated that she was blessed to have such a good man who does so much for others. Her friends all agreed. Sharon said nothing more; she had learned from Nate that bragging should never be done. Marjorie thought it could be disrespectful; Nate agreed. Sharon would savor these compliments by herself.

Sharon knew that she really did like helping people. Many times Sharon saw that when she helped one of the adults in town, their faces lit up with joy. Subsequently, Sharon's heart lit up in the same way. She loved the feeling. Sharon could never forget the happiness and joy in a child's face after she did something for them. She had experienced this countless times with Lizzie and Ruthie. It never got old. Sharon thoroughly cherished that the joy and happiness between the three had grown into the best emotion – love.

She thought her desire to help was partly because of two reasons. One was that she couldn't help for most of her life because she didn't have anything to give. Sharon struggled to survive, both physically and emotionally. Later in life, she did manage to give out a jar of jam occasionally but had to be careful that her husband didn't find out. Many people guessed that Sharon was relatively poor. The other reason she wanted to help was that no one helped her when she was a child. She was hungry and cold too many times growing up. Sharon never forgot this. She was dedicated to helping children. Luckily, she had a husband who agreed with everything she did.

Mrs. Johnson had developed into a new person since meeting Nate; the whole town knew it. Nate told Sharon that all the goodness and kindness were always there inside her heart; they just had to be let out. He was glad to help because he loved her from the first time they hugged. Nate mentioned in one of their talks that he believed that women have a more caring soul than men do. God has given women the wherewithal to take care of babies and young children. Sharon mentioned that her wonderful husband is patient and caring. The response was, "Most men do care to some degree; it's hard to put a number on it. Let us just say women care more. I care a great deal about helping children, but you, my dear, caring, and lovable wife, are better. In fact, you are the most caring person I know. It is one of the many reasons why I love you so much." Those words were followed by a long hug and kiss.

Sharon knew that she valued people, not just her friends, but also everybody she met. It didn't matter if you were rich or poor, skilled or unskilled, man or woman, old or young. She had the same feeling for all nationalities. Everybody has value and should be appreciated and respected. Mrs. Johnson was always pleasant and kind. Her smiles and friendly mannerisms made people comfortable talking with her. Everyone sensed that she cared about them. She knew that Marjorie was the same way. Nate never forgot the first Friday the two cowboys who guarded the herd came for their 36 hours off. The hot water was ready; dinner was being prepared. Sharon treated the men like friends. She and Nate joined the men at the barbeque to enjoy the fire, food, and good conversation. The men told Nate, later, that Sharon was the nicest person they had ever known. Nate thanked them as he shook their hands and said, "There are many folks who say the same thing."

Mary, Jeremy, and Andy were very happy living in the new town. It had taken them about a year to make the move. The Johnsons really valued their first three years in their new setting. It was great being close to family. They loved the new opportunities this place afforded them. The Moores had built a rather large addition onto Sharon's place for the twins. Andy loved the spaciousness of the room. He even invited a couple of friends over to study and have lunch several times. He was doing well in his studies and enjoyed the independent style of the upper grades. He did the work at his pace and reported in to several teachers. Thomas, Dan, and Betty were still helping with the upper grades. It wasn't long before Jeremy and Mary were also assisting.

Andy enjoyed the new school. He strongly felt that the girls were the best part. Andy had made the normal transition that young boys make from girl haters to big fans of the female persuasion. He was almost eighteen now. He actually had his eye on one young woman in particular. Andy liked everything about this new town. He was learning more outside of school than in. He really liked that.

Doris was married and expecting. She had married a college professor when she was almost twenty-two. Mac Jones was twenty-four when the couple married. He had been a history professor for two years. He was a very popular instructor with a bright future. Doris had taken a class from Mac. They met after he gave Doris an A- on a paper. After their discussion, he changed the grade to an A. She had been right in her assessment. Mac was very impressed. The couple was a perfect match; they couldn't be any happier. Doris was tutoring part time. The Johnsons at the JT Ranch missed Doris, but they understood the couple's desire to stay where the jobs were. Doris had become a city girl; she loved what it had to offer. She loved Mac even more.

With all the children virtually grown up, Mary had some time on her hands. She had always enjoyed sewing. It could be a creative activity. This was something that Mary naturally gravitated towards. She had a mind that liked to create, whether it was poetry; new dishes for family dinners, or, in the past, lesson plans for the students. She was really enjoying teaching the older students. Dan noticed how talented she was. In a short time, he started to cut his time in the classroom. The students would benefit from Mary much more than from him. He knew that he was a good teacher. Mary was just better. He felt no shame in stepping down over time.

The talented Jeremy enjoyed not having the pressure from having to write and deliver the Sunday sermon. He was free to build furniture. He and Thomas loved working and visiting together. They constructed wonderful pieces. Jeremy also enjoyed doing some chores around the ranch. He and Nate would sometimes go on an afternoon ride. It never got old to see such beautiful countryside. The older Johnsons, with Sharon's permission, named her old place Small Ranch. Jeremy even made a sign. Sharon and Nate loved it.

Thomas and Dee seemed very happy. They had been married for about three years. The couple's favorite activity was cooking. An activity allowed them to talk, laugh, and sample the food they were preparing. Thomas still liked to work; he visited the JT or the Small Ranch almost every day. He visited the cattle often, tended to the horses, and worked with Jeremy and Nate. Sometimes Andy would join in, and that was fun to see.

Dr. Smith was still the town's minister. He and Dee wrote the sermons together. They both really enjoyed the activity. Dee was a great writer and knew the Bible as well as Thomas. People were still praising the talented minister. Thomas gave all the credit for the new sermons to Dee. He wanted everyone to appreciate her as much as he did. Both were around sixty years old. They both leaned on the other when they needed to. Sharon had seen it a couple of times and thought it was better than wonderful. IT TOUCHED HER HEART.

Nate and Sharon were talking about family one night when Nate said, with a smile on his face, that their horse family had grown by two. He added that it is hard to count the increase in the cattle family. Sharon took Nate's hands and squeezed them three times. She said, "There's no doubt that the financial aspect of the JT Ranch is doing very well. I am very happy about the business of the ranch. I am excited about our growth of family. Locally, we have gone from three to twelve. I love it; I'm sure you do too." The couple hugged for a long time. Shortly, their family would grow again.

Chapter 17

New Arrivals

One Saturday afternoon, a strange looking wagon pulled into town. Nate and Sharon were taking the best minister in town and his lovely wife out to an early dinner to celebrate Thomas' sixty-second birthday. They all saw the wagon but paid little attention to it. They were preoccupied with the joyous celebration. Nate suggested that he lead a toast with everyone having a glass of wine.

Thomas started laughing and said, "You two go to sleep almost immediately after having a glass. Unless there's a bed in the back of the restaurant, I suggest we toast with water." Everybody laughed; they all knew it was true.

Nate did propose a toast to his mentor. He explained that he had never given a toast before, but he had eaten many slices. Everyone smiled. The thirty year old told the others that he once was told to follow his heart. He did, and the words that followed were heartfelt and touching. He ended with the words that he wanted to shake the hand of the greatest man he had ever known. Thomas stood up, shook Nate's hand rather robustly, and for the third time in eight years gave his "son" a hearty hug.

From where Sharon was sitting in the restaurant, she could see down the street. As she listened to Nate, she saw six children, the driver, and a man in a suit exit a wagon. She squeezed her husband's hand three times to let him know that she loved him and his words. Sharon continued to watch as the man in the suit entered the restaurant and started talking to the host. After Nate finished his words and embrace with his mentor, Sharon saw the man starting to leave the eatery. She quickly excused herself from the table, explaining that she would be right back. She told Nate to order her usual.

Mrs. Johnson caught the man at the wagon as he was talking to the others. She quickly smiled and introduced herself. Sharon added that the man sure had some well-behaved children. She couldn't wait for his reply. Sharon smiled; squatted down, and shook the two little girls' hands. Sharon continued to hold their hands as she told them it was a joy to meet them. She also shook the little boy's hand, smiled again, and said similar words to him.

Mr. Avery introduced himself as Sharon stood back up, "These children are orphans. They are in my care. We're traveling down the road about twenty miles where the children may be adopted." He mentioned that they had stopped for dinner and a place to spend the night, but the prices were too high. Sharon quickly surmised that this was a kind and caring man. Mr. Avery continued, "The children will have a snack and sleep in the wagon. We've all done this before."

Mrs. Johnson told Mr. Avery, "My husband and I would love to buy your whole crew dinner. My husband has money in his pocket; it is starting to burn a hole in his pants. He needs to spend it quickly, or I will have to mend his pocket. You would be doing me a huge favor by letting him buy you dinner." Sharon was smiling most of the time as she spoke. She could tell the three older boys and the two adults enjoyed her words; they were all smiling. The younger fourth boy was holding hands with two smaller girls. Sharon thought they were listening but noticed there was no change in their expressions.

The "crew" entered the restaurant. The one large table just happened to be available. Sharon accompanied the group and host to the table. Nate saw what was happening and joined them as they were sitting down. He introduced himself saying that he was the husband of this wonderful woman who warms his heart every day. Sharon smiled and told her Nate that he was buying these wonderful people dinner. Mr. Johnson said, "It's our pleasure to do so. I always like it when my wife makes new friends." He added that the steak is wonderful as is the spaghetti. Luckily, Nate had extra cash in his wallet.

He went back to the birthday celebration. Sharon stayed behind to visit briefly with the children. She was somewhat concerned about the two little girls. Mrs. Johnson looked amazing; she was dressed in one of Michelle's great creations. She had on her expensive dress cowboy boots purchased by her loving husband and some very pretty accessories that were gifts from Thomas and Dee. Her last birthday had been very special. Sharon was telling the children what meals were some of the local favorites. She also mentioned the desserts. She finished up as the server arrived. The cowgirl told Mr. Avery that the group would be more than welcome to stay at the JT Ranch. There are three bedrooms and three couches at your disposal. There is a corral for the horses and plenty of feed and water. She exited after telling the group to take their time and enjoy their dinner. The two adults and the three older boys smiled and thanked her. The fourth boy thanked her but with no smile. There was no response from the little girls. This really bothered Sharon.

Sharon apologized to the Smiths and her husband for interrupting Thomas' special day. Thomas laughed and said, "I've had sixty-two of these days; they are not that special anymore. Dee and I agree that watching you help a group in need is way beyond special." Nate chipped in with words about her kindness. He took her hand as he was speaking and squeezed it three times. Sharon thanked the men for their wonderful words. She also said that Dee would have done the same if she had seen the wagon on the street. Dee smiled at that thoughtful comment.

Sharon mentioned to Nate that she might have overstepped. She invited the whole crew out to the ranch to spend the night. The husband of this kind and loving woman smiled, leaned over, kissed her on the cheek, and explained that he would have been disappointed if she had not invited the group. Thomas and Dee just sat there and smiled.

The two buggies and the large wagon made their way out to the JT Ranch. Mr. Avery was very impressed with everything, but he did not say anything. He had learned in his business to let the others do the talking. He could get a better read on people that way. He had been in the orphanage business pretty much his whole life. He was orphaned at the age of five and grew up in three different orphanages. He worked at the last place when he turned eighteen. He continued to advance in the business until he reached his current level. He had a passion for placing children into the best possible scenario. It wasn't always easy. There was constant pressure to put children into private homes even if they weren't always a great choice. Boys were always easier to place because they became good farm or ranch hands. Girls weren't as popular. He was worried about the three little ones.

As everybody stretched their legs after sitting for so long, the visitors got a chance to see the immediate surroundings. All of them were very impressed. Mr. Avery had been to many homes. This was, rapidly, the best one he had ever seen. As the entire group of twelve walked around, a group of seven soon approached them.

Sharon and Nate quickly approached Nate's parents, as the younger Johnsons had not seen Mary and Jeremy for eight days. They had been to Chicago to visit their new grandchild. They also hadn't seen Andy all week. He had been so busy with work. Mr. Avery observed the hellos between the five. There were hugs, handshakes, and many smiles accompanied by some kind words. The keen-eyed visitor was impressed.

Mr. Avery watched as the ranch owners said their greetings to the four people who had stayed back aways. These four had work clothes on. Mr. Avery guessed that they were employees of the ranch, but the words and smiles indicated something different. The observant administrator took note that Mrs. Johnson was a very friendly person.

Mrs. Johnson made all the introductions. Nate couldn't believe that his wife remembered all the names of all eight visitors. She told everybody that since the whole bunch is going to be friends, first names are necessary. Sharon spent a moment talking about each member of the Johnson family; it was a nice touch. She told the visitors, "Jeremy is a retired minister; he now makes amazing furniture and helps out here at the JT. Mary was a teacher in the past; she still teaches me many things. Andy has worked in the local store for four years; he and his fiancé are in the process of buying it."

Sharon walked over near John and explained to the guests, "John and his two daughters, Elizabeth and Ruthie, are family. John helps us here on the ranch; the girls are very helpful with chores. They also have a riding school for children and a horse rental business. This nice looking young man is Lizzie's friend, Steve. He lives on a ranch nearby. He helps the girls run the two businesses." Mr. Avery couldn't believe how pleasant everyone was. He liked being introduced as Allen; it was a friendly gesture. Allen had previously had a brief talk with Thomas and Dee. He found out that the animal doctor had known Nate for almost his entire life. The vet and Dee also said they were family.

The orphanage administrator wondered if Nate and Sharon were looking to adopt. He loved the extended family. This was so nice for orphans to be part of. Large families provide a variety of events that allow the orphans a greater chance to join in and become comfortable. This happens less than 50% of the time. Sharon and Nate demonstrated great skills with children. He loved how Lizzie and Ruthie had both squatted down to hug Susan and Sally. They shook Sammy's hand, smiled, and said how nice it was to meet him. He actually smiled back. Mr. Avery knew who taught Lizzie and Ruthie to be so kind. The headman of the orphanage was very impressed with Mrs. Johnson.

Allen and his assistant, Henry, walked around the property with Thomas; it was Thomas' idea. Thomas told the men, "Nate and Sharon have a gift with children, but they won't ask about Sammy, Sally, and Susan because they wouldn't want to put you in a predicament. It also wouldn't be right to interfere with the arranged visit that is forthcoming." The vet asked

Allen to please remember that the three little ones would be readily adopted if Nate and Sharon were asked to care for the children. Allen informed Thomas that the couple in question twenty miles away is not a sure thing to take all three. They only want Sammy, but they were convinced to consider all three. The children do not want to be split up. Thomas thanked the men for their time.

Lizzie and Ruthie took the little ones to see all the animals while the three older boys played games with Andy. Steve had excused himself earlier as he was due home. The Jacob girls were fantastic with their guests. It was the first time Allen saw the three little ones smile in a long time. Allen walked over to John to tell him how wonderful his daughters were. Mr. Avery thanked John for having such nice daughters who would spend time playing with visitors.

John asked Allen to please follow him. As they walked away, Mr. Jacobs explained, "I absolutely love Nate and Sharon." He told Allen that his wife died several years ago. When Sharon found out, she quickly befriended us. "I couldn't possibly repay the Johnsons for what they have done. The first thing Sharon did was lend me a buggy and horse to ride out to the JT. Nate gave me a job. They both knew I was always looking for income to help take care of the girls. Sharon also knew that I needed help with my girls. I was overwhelmed with all the responsibility. In a very short time, Sharon asked me to bring the girls out for breakfast. She also mentioned how much fun it would be to have five people to visit with during breakfast. My workload quickly grew to five or six days a week at the ranch with Sharon and Nate helping with my girls. They are both truly wonderful with Lizzie and Ruthie. My kids love them dearly." John's eyes had watered up some.

Mr. Avery thanked John for the information. He had made his decision. Sammy, Susan, and Sally would stay with Nate and Sharon if the couple asked that it be so. Allen would talk to Thomas; he seemed to know everybody and definitely was close to Nate and Sharon.

Allen always kept adoption papers in his briefcase. There was no doubt that the Johnsons had enough references. The server at the restaurant told Mr. Avery that he had just met the most amazing couple in town; everybody thinks the world of them. The administrator would tell the couple he was scheduled to see tomorrow that he placed Sammy. Susan, and Sally into a home in town. There was a doctor in the family, and the girls needed some special looking after. Allen would say how sorry he was, but he had not known about the girls' condition until after making the introduction plans with them. He would apologize again and explain that the children are his responsibility. He must always, by law, place them in the best situation possible. He would find them a replacement as soon as possible, a bigger and older boy than Sammy.

Mr. Avery approached Thomas and Dee. He asked if he might have a word with them. He explained, "The cart seems to be in front of the horse in this situation, but I want the three smaller children to be adopted by Nate and Sharon. I have never done anything like this before; it is all backwards. There is supposed to be an application along with three references, which are all verified. I then approve the paperwork and send it to the proper authorities to be legally approved. Nate and Sharon finish the process by signing the documents in front of an officer of the court. I have never had a situation where I initiated the adoption, but here I am, doing just that. There is a stipulation in the adoption process that allows local clergy to provide care for the children until the paperwork is complete. Steve mentioned to me that you and Jeremy are ministers."

Thomas told Allen, "It looks like you need a few things from me. I am sure I can help. I will go talk to Nate and Sharon immediately. I know their answer already, but let me make it official. The rest we will discuss as soon as I get back. I am so excited for them."

Thomas had a big smile on his face as he approached Nate and Sharon, who were talking to Nate's parents. He quickly asked if he could talk to the younger couple in private.

Mary and Jeremy walked off to visit elsewhere. They spotted Andy and Bethany talking. She had just pulled up in her family's buggy.

After the personable vet asked his question about the children, Sharon's response spoke volumes about what kind of team Nate and Sharon were. She took Nate's hand and said that they have so much to share. She then asked what he thought. He responded, "We have a loving, kind, and supporting family. The children would be blessed to have such a family. What do you want to do, my lovely wife?"

"Let's ask our family what they think, and then we can take a walk to discuss it," said a smiling Sharon.

As the family was gathering per Sharon's request, Nate was asking Mr. Avery and his crew if they could please walk out to see the lumber mill for a few minutes. Mr. Avery knew exactly what was going on. He quickly agreed to Nate's request. Thomas had gone over to bring Dee to the group. He informed her as they slowly walked to the group that Nate and Sharon had not mentioned one word about the cost, time, or work in taking the kids. They only talked about how good it would be for the children. He said, "Giving this ranch to Nate and Sharon has made me so proud. My good deed has been multiplied a number of times. Today is their greatest deed so far. There will be many more."

Sharon was the one to address the group. She told everybody that something big might be happening, and she and Nate needed the family is input. John wasn't sure if he was family enough to be involved in any big decisions, but he knew that his daughters thought of themselves as full-fledged members of the Johnson clan. Sharon explained to the group that she and Nate have been given the opportunity to adopt Sammy, Susan, and Sally. She finished with the words, "We won't move forward unless you agree."

Mary knew immediately that Sharon was using the same tactic that she had used in moving here. M2 also knew that adopting the children was the absolute right call. These children would be loved, supported, and grow to be something special. She glanced at Andy and Jeremy who gave her quick nods. Mary told the group. "My family is 100% behind the adoption. Not only do we think Nate and Sharon would be fantastic parents, we will do whatever we can to further the love and support for these wonderful children. This is a blessing from God." She was crying.

John Jacobs spoke next, "We love the idea of adopting the three children. We, like the elder Johnsons, will do whatever we can for the new additions to our family." Sharon was thrilled that he had said "our family".

Thomas said that he had so many words to say that he could not possibly say them all now. "I will speak at a later date, but for now, we say that this adoption is a marvelous idea. We are totally aboard with everything."

Two minutes later, when Mr. Avery and his crew returned, Thomas was nodding his head. Sharon and Nate had only taken a thirty-second walk. When Thomas saw Sharon jumping up and down a couple of times, he knew the couple's decision. Mr. Avery asked Sharon and Nate if they wanted to tell Sammy, Susan, and Sally something?

Sharon and Nate held hands as Sharon spoke "Will you wonderful children, Sammy,

Susan, and Sally, let Nate and I adopt you?"

Sally, the six year old, started running towards Sharon. Mrs. Johnson quickly squatted down. In a split second, Susan joined the hug between Sharon and Sally. Nate squatted down with his wife and was joined in a hug with Sammy. The children swapped places and the hugging continued. Everybody was so thrilled for the children and the married couple. Sharon was crying some because she could not contain the joy in her heart. Mary had a few more tears as she whispered a "thank you" to M. The three older orphan boys, Matt, Joey, and Robert, had watery eyes; they were so happy for their orphanage mates.

The children went back to playing while Allen and Henry walked back together to get some paperwork for the adoption. Henry had also grown up in an orphanage. After reaching legal age, he became a repairperson on the grounds. He explained to his friend that he loved Nate and Sharon adopting the children. Both men agreed that it was a perfect fit. Henry stated, "All of this would not have happened if you hadn't wanted to stop at the restaurant. You normally visit the sheriff's office first to ask for advice. Why didn't you go there?"

"I just had a feeling. I went with it," said the boss. "Henry, I don't believe I've ever been so happy about an adoption." Henry agreed.

A short time later, Thomas, Dee, and Mr. Avery started talking about the paperwork on the way to the Smith house. Allen explained it all; it wasn't very difficult. Mr. Avery told the Smiths that he and

Henry would be coming back through town on Monday in the early evening. The administrator mentioned that usually the biggest obstacles are the signatures by a local official and an officer of the court. Thomas smiled and stated that this wouldn't be a problem in this instance. He told Allen that all the paperwork would be completed by noon on Monday. He added that these three children are so fortunate to have such a fantastic family. Henry and Allen completely agreed.

Sharon and Nate told Thomas on Saturday that they wouldn't be in church on Sunday. The Jacobs were coming over for breakfast. Sharon wanted the five children to get better acquainted. She didn't want to overwhelm Sammy, Susan, and Sally with herself and Nate. Mrs. Johnson thought there would be plenty of conversation before breakfast. Nate and Sharon would involve all six new arrivals in the preparation of the breakfast. During and after breakfast Lizzie and Ruthie would take over. This would give the new Johnsons a time to play and converse with their "cousins".

Nate loved his wife's thoughts. Don't take a chance of smothering and let the children be kids playing with kids. Sharon's gift with children was shining bright. There was no doubt who was going to be in charge when it came to the children. Nate would assist and support his amazing wife's ideas and whatever direction she thought was correct. He also knew that every night the two loving parents would talk and share thoughts about their new family members.

All five children thoroughly enjoyed their time together. The little ones were actually smiling, laughing, and interacting with Lizzle and Ruthie. Allen and Henry had picked up the older boys right after breakfast. Nate, Sharon, and John spent some time watching the five play. John mentioned to the Johnsons that they had done a marvelous job in making his daughters so loving and kind. Nate simply said that they had the greatest role model to follow. He squeezed Sharon's hand three times.

It was decided that the Jacobs would go home midafternoon. Sharon and Nate would take charge at that time. There had been ample interaction between the five actual Johnson family members during the day. John went for a hike after lunch; this allowed Nate and Sharon to focus on the children. Nate played a few games with them with Sharon as the cheerleader. It was extremely pleasant for everyone, especially Sharon.

Just as the Jacobs were getting ready to leave, Sharon wanted to ask the children a few questions. She had already talked with Nate about what she was about to propose. Mrs. Johnson explained that Lizzie does much of her schoolwork here at the JT. She doesn't go to school every day, but Ruthie does. Grandma Mary and Lizzie would love to talk to Susan and Sally about school and do a few lessons. Ruthie will take Sammy to school as they are in the same grade. She could introduce him to everybody. Sharon asked if Sammy and the girls would agree to this plan. She added that she absolutely loved Ruthie for being so kind. She also liked the idea that our girls get to meet Nate's mother, who is more than wonderful. The children all agreed to the plan; Nate knew they would. Nobody could say no to the woman with the friendly smile.

It was Sharon's plan for Ruthie to take care of Sammy at school for at least a day. Everybody very well liked Ruthie. She could really help the situation. Once Sammy was comfortable, Sharon and Nate would take the girls to school. They seemed somewhat fragile, especially Sally. Mary could help with a few lessons to get a gauge on the girls.

The girls would go to school when they were ready. The little ones were opening up to

Lizzie and Ruthie with some smiles and laughing. They seemed to enjoy their new parents. Sharon and Nate wanted a smooth transition into school. There was no need to rush.

Andy and Bethany's wedding was four weeks away. The couple became involved while working at the store. Andy had started work there at sixteen; he loved the job. He was a very friendly person. In no time, he knew all the regular customer's names and enjoyed visiting as he was assisting them. Bethany started working at the store six months after Andy. Her father was the local doctor. He did not like her taking the job at all, but Beth would not be denied. She had a huge crush on Andy. The two teenagers were soon seeing each other. At Bethany's house, the visits were quite formal; usually Beth's mother attended. The couple didn't care; they finished all their studies working together. Both were bright; Beth had privately asked their teachers if they could tie for the top honors in school. She thought that would be cute.

Andy talked to Thomas after graduation one day about the storeowner. Andy said the owner wasn't doing as well as he was two years ago. Dr. Smith explained it could be all the alcohol the storeowner has consumed over the years. Some people can drink for years with very little effect, but others will show decreased mental capacity along with less energy. Medical science doesn't know why this happens, but it does. Andy told Thomas that this information explains exactly what he has seen at work. The store clerk also told the senior member of the Johnson family that the store stocks one type of whiskey. Nobody seems to ever buy it, but the store orders a case every month.

The kind vet told Andy, "If you like the work, learn as much as you can about it. You might have a chance to buy the business. It just might be a great opportunity. The people of this town need a well-run store. Dan Perkins would be the man to talk to if that time ever occurs."

In the next year, Andy and Bethany took over so much of the running of the store that they decided to talk to Dan. Dan, of course, knew of the situation; most people in town did. The storeowner's knees and shoulders hurt often. They were the results of a saloon life that had gotten physical in his younger days, not to mention the numerous falls. He was getting forgetful. Everyone knew the young couple was running the store.

Dan told the engaged couple that he would talk to the owner on their behalf. It will be your wedding present. Andy and Beth thanked him so much for his help. They were thrilled with the prospect of running their own business. Dan loved helping anyone in the

Johnson family. It was a small payment compared to what the family had done for this town.

Andy and Bethany decided to have a small wedding. If they invited several customer friends, other customers might feel left out. Bethany's dad wanted some of his out of town business friends invited. The couple did not want that. Bethany's mother, Barbara, was caught in the middle. A simple solution was to have Mary, Sharon, and Barbara handle all the arrangements. Dr. Melvin Hemfield was not happy that the wedding reception was going to take place at the JT Ranch. He liked being in charge calling all the shots, but he knew Bethany didn't want either of those things.

The three women, along with input from the engaged couple, planned all the details. It didn't take long for Barbara to become a fan of Mary and Sharon. The wedding itself was going to be somewhat formal. Both Thomas and Jeremy would speak; Jeremy would provide the actual service. Thomas' words would bring joy to the occasion. All five of the wedding planners thought this was a great idea. It would add a very special touch to the ceremony. It might even make Dr. Hemfield smile.

There were going to be four flower girls and a ring bearer. Susan and Sally were excited to be walking down the aisle with Lizzie and Ruthie. The four were growing very close. Sammy thought he had a very important job. Lizzie wanted to make her and Ruthie's dress; Sharon and Mary would assist. Mary was making the little girls' dresses; they both were very excited about it. Mary was so good at sewing. She continued to teach Sharon advanced skills every so often. The three Hemfields had picked out Bethany's dress earlier. Bethany thought her father would be happy that he had a hand in picking out the dress. He would also enjoy paying for it. The bride knew he would mention to everybody that he picked out the dress and paid for it.

The wedding went very well. Everybody loved the flower girls and the ring bearer, and the church looked great. Everybody was in a festive mood as they headed back to the JT for the reception. This was where Andy and Bethany wanted the celebration to be. The men had cleared out some of the furniture for a dance floor. Sharon had mentioned to Nate years ago that their living room was big enough to hold a party in. She sometimes would call it the "great room". It was splendid. The men were able to set two large dining room tables and chairs off to one side. They would move them out on the dance floor when dinner was ready and put them together. All sixteen people would sit at one rather large table. The bride and groom loved it. The main cooks, Thomas and Dee, along with their helpers, Mary and Sharon, put out snacks while completing the final changes on the dinner.

Bethany's only concern was her father. He had insisted before the wedding on purchasing several bottles of champagne in order to give a proper toast. He was already drinking. His daughter knew that sometimes-inappropriate words came out of his mouth after a few drinks. She saw her mother preparing the glasses. All Bethany could do was to hope for the best. Dr. Hemfield told everyone to grab a glass because he wanted to propose a toast to the newlyweds. His only child held her breath as he said, "I toast the bride and groom. As you all know, I am a member of the grandest profession, the medical field. I wanted my daughter to join me as an invaluable partner, but she chose, instead, to work in a store. Good luck to them both at the store." The insinuation was not enjoyed by anyone.

As everybody took a polite sip, Thomas quickly added, "I also have a toast. I believe we have all had the privilege of seeing this wonderful couple working together. Don't you just love it? Dee and I have had many conversations about how happy they are. Seeing them together in the store puts any observer in a better mood. I think that is fantastic. Andy and Bethany, please continue to provide an invaluable resource to the community. I know you will always make people smile when they see you together." "Here here" was the response of almost all of the adults, including Barbara.

Nate had the misfortune to be standing next to Melvin when he and Thomas proposed their very different toasts. Dr. Hemfield had cornered Nate in conversation. Nate was being polite in making small talk. He was nervously sipping on the champagne. When the glass was half-empty, Melvin filled it. The conversation went on until

Sharon rescued her husband, explaining to the doctor that Nate's muscles were needed in the kitchen.

As they entered the kitchen, Mary was standing right there. All the food was ready; there was nothing left to do. Mary had sent her daughter-in-law to the rescue. It was twenty minutes to dinner, and Mary had observed Nate is drinking. She also knew that he wasn't a drinker. She and Jeremy had taken a sip and poured the rest out in the kitchen. Before she could talk, Nate made the following statement. "Boy that was a dumb toast by Dr. Hemfield."

Mary shot her son a stern look; Nate saw it. Before he could say anything, Sharon stated that she heard it. She quickly mentioned to her husband that she needed some fresh air. Would her fantastic husband like to join her? Nate said that it would be his pleasure. They held hands as they walked outside. "J, you know that I love you more than words can describe, right?" said Sharon.

As Nate embraced his wife, he told her, "T, thank you for saying that. We have been quite busy for the last month; each day I still love our time. It has been cut short a number of times because Sally and Susan have visited us in our room at night, but I would not change a thing. I love it when they come in. When we walked out here holding hands, it just fills me with joy. So, our alone time may be somewhat less than before, but each second now means more to me than before."

Sharon kissed her husband, and said she wanted to share some thoughts with her brilliant husband. She went on to explain that this reception today is to celebrate Andy and Bethany's marriage. It should be all about them. It should be great fun and very positive in all aspects, especially spoken words. Dr. Hemfield was very wrong in his toast. Nobody liked it; it dampened the mood immediately. Bethany's facial expression demonstrated anger. There was not a smile in the whole room. Luckily, Thomas jumped in with his touching words. He brought back the good thoughts about the newlyweds and the joy of the occasion. This reception should only be filled with smiles. Laughs and all things positive.

At that moment as Sharon was finishing her words, Mary brought her son a cup of coffee. She told Nate that she was very aware that he did not drink coffee in the early evenings, but tonight might be an exception. She said that dinner was in fifteen minutes. She left.

Nate stated that his mother was not happy. Sharon agreed with her husband's assessment. Nate started drinking the coffee; Sharon was rubbing his other hand. She wasn't speaking. Nate looked out at the surroundings, away from Sharon. He kept drinking the coffee. He was starting to put it together. Dr. Hemfield was wrong with his words. Nate knew he was also wrong. His words were not positive and supportive; they definitely weren't joyous and happy. If he had said them to somebody out in the great room, he might have done some real damage.

The father of three thanked his wife for the lesson on celebrations. He said that he will never forget her words. Nate then asked his wife if she could bring his mother out for a second. Mary and Sharon reappeared in less than a minute. They were holding hands. Nate thought that was a good sign. He didn't have to apologize often, but he did now.

Nate told his mother, "Many things started going through my mind after I came outside. Your lessons about kindness and love started reverberating inside my head. M's lessons about salons and oral communication resurfaced in my brain. I said something that was totally wrong. My very smart wife just taught a lesson about celebrations that I will never forget. Mother, I am so sorry that I disappointed you. It will never happen again. This mistake is not who I am as a Johnson clan member."

Mary simply said, "You made a mistake. Sometimes that is how we learn. You could have caused some serious damage to the festivities tonight, but, luckily, your negative comments were only heard by two people who absolutely know those words are not the Nate Johnson that we love and adore." She gave her son an extended hug and told the couple that dinner was in five minutes.

Sharon mentioned to Nate, "I am so proud of my wonderful husband. Being a Johnson clan member makes me a better person. You, M2, and Thomas have taught this little farm girl so much about life." She had been hugging him and continued doing so while she finished her words by saying, "My kind and loving husband has filled me with so much joy. I couldn't be any happier."

The couple walked into the house holding hands. Nate knew exactly what his wife had just done. When a mistake is made involving them, the person making the mistake issues a heartfelt apology; positive words of support come from the other person. There is always some sign of affection, and then it is never discussed again. He squeezed his wife's hand three times.

Thomas, Mary, and Sharon led the conversation at the wonderful feast. They all were full of praises for the newlyweds. There were many smiles and a few laughs. Mary told a cute story about Andy when he had just turned three. They were shopping in the store. Andy had "helped" himself to a couple of jellybeans. She could only hope that Bethany could control him now that he is the co-owner of a grocery store. Everybody laughed at the story.

Some started kidding him about being a lawbreaker. Bethany said that while they are in the store, she allows Andy one jellybean after a hug and kiss. Andy smiled and said, "I always win. A crowded store means we are making money; an empty store means I can hug and kiss my lovely Beth and have a jellybean. Sometimes she even lets me pick out my favorite flavor." As he said these last words, he reached over and took Bethany's hand. Everybody saw the love and joy between the two.

After dinner, Nate made it a point to visit with Dr. Hem field. He wanted to be positive and pleasant during the conversation. The doctor had been quiet during dinner. He was standing by himself as Nate approached. The co-owner of the JT shook the doctor's hand while telling him it must be a great feeling to have such fine skills and knowledge. The conversation continued with Nate talking about doing good deeds and being a positive influence. Dr. Hemfield thought Nate was talking about him until the skilled blacksmith said that everybody in this room is a blessing for what they do for others.

As the reception was ending, Nate went outside to think for a few minutes. He definitely had something to talk to Sharon about, not tonight, but maybe in a couple of days. He was outside when the bride and groom were making their exit to go back into town where their new home was waiting for them. Mary and Sharon had done a few special things to decorate the house. There were even a few snacks, including a couple of jellybeans.

Chapter 18

More Jobs

Dan Perkins and Colonel Jones were in the process of bringing new jobs to town. The Colonel was retired now and wanted everybody to call him Rich or Richard. Rich and Dan were business partners. The Colonel had never married and did not have any family back East. He liked Dan's town and decided to explore his opportunities. Dan and Rich had been good friends for quite a while. They had great respect for each other and enjoyed talking about the history of the United States. Dan knew the town very well and the Colonel had a sharp logical mind. Together they planned and executed endeavors that were profitable, along with adding employment opportunities for the younger people of the town. The pair loved bringing new jobs to town.

The fort Rich was stationed at for Major Roger Haynes was now leading quite a few years. Dan and Rich were so proud of Roger's performance. He had gone up the ranks rather quickly, deservedly so. The army was building a new fort 100 miles to the southwest. Most of the men currently under Major Hayne's command would be reassigned to the new location. The Major would accompany his men. All the soldiers thought so highly of this fine officer. He would be in command of the new larger fort that housed a complete company of troops. Rich promised to visit during the construction. He would be the only one allowed to call the Major by his given name. Everybody else would call him Lt. Colonel Haynes, Colonel for short.

The army wanted the fort to provide additional security for the railroad construction. Because there were still occasional problems towards the west, there was a need for the army's presence. Dan and Rich had already talked to Nate about increasing production at the JT lumber mill. The lumber mill at the current fort had closed as the owners had exhausted the supply of trees. Dan and Rich accomplished two smart business moves, buy 10,000 acres of prime timberland southwest of the JT Ranch and purchase the now closed sawmill near the fort. Neither deal was very costly. The two men thought they could create a number of jobs and make a few dollars at the same time.

Nate and Sharon told John Jacobs what Lt. Colonel Haynes needed in terms of lumber for the fort; the dimensions were also given. There was a discussion of how many men to hire. It was decided that four men would be added to bring logs to the mill and two more to help around the mill. John was excited because Rich had also mentioned raising the price of the lumber. Sharon was thrilled because she and the girls could plant more trees.

Sharon and her crew always planted two trees for each one cut down. She told the girls they were building homes for the squirrels and birds. They loved that thought.

Nate and Sharon hired more people to help the JT in various capacities. Two ranch hands did a little bit of everything at the boarding house, Small Ranch, and at the JT. Nate supervised the men. Jam and jerky sales created more jobs with Sharon in charge. JT Jerky was a popular local product. Nancy had left a very tasty recipe, and after Nate and Sharon made the first batch of the spicy treat, they knew they had something special. Sales of jam and jerky went up on a yearly basis, but, lately, there was a substantial increase. Major Haynes was the person responsible for the dramatic increase.

Every week an army wagon or two would travel to Dodge City for supplies. The Major thought it was silly to take an empty wagon for supplies. Why not fill it with some local goods? The army would charge a small fee for the transportation. It would be great for everybody. The Major was a big fan of all the local products. Some were very original; others entailed unique workmanship. He especially liked the bird houses and several flavors of jams. Sharon had shared Nancy's jam recipe with a few women. Jam was a source of revenue for several families in town. The town appreciated the Major's help in selling their wares. Occasionally, Jeremy's furniture and/or birdhouses found their way on the wagon.

Andy and Bethany were also connected to the plan. Andy had talked to the Major about buying staples in bulk for the fort and the two area stores. Buying in bulk would save money and make the items more profitable. Major Haynes really liked Andy's idea. He drafted a letter to the broker in Topeka who agreed to the deal. The Major really liked the owners of Beth's Store, a place he used to help protect. The Major still had fond memories of his work at the outpost. The people of the town had been very appreciative of the army's presence. The officer always enjoyed visiting with the civilians during the town markets. He knew many – from young to old. The Major still considered many of them as friends.

The outpost had been closed since Colonel Jone's retirement. Thomas decided that he would make it into a boarding house for single workers. Before the outpost was even functioning, Dr. Smith had purchased all the kitchen appliances, all the bedding needs, and enough furniture to equip the entire place, including the office. Now the place was empty. There was definitely a need for cheap housing for the young unmarried men of the town, and he just happened to have a place to offer. He also hired two young women to cook and tend to the area during the day. The occupants of the house would watch over the place at night. The outpost was still being used twice a month for town markets and once a month for the town dinner and dance. It was very important to keep the place looking good.

Andy and Bethany were in their last year of paying off the store. They had upgraded the interior of the store, thus creating more space for products. It was done section by section with Nate, Thomas, and Jeremy doing all the work. The three skilled workers also made a fine shed to house canned items that had been purchased in bulk. The men had a great time working together.

One pleasant Sunday afternoon, Sharon approached Andy and Beth at a family gathering at the JT. She explained that she and Nate wanted to know if the younger Johnsons had ever considered opening a line of credit for some customers. Andy and Beth were very aware that income was often seasonal. They always felt terrible to see some people counting their money to see if they had enough for the items they were purchasing, especially young couples with small children. Andy and Beth always did their best to help if it was only a few cents.

Sharon said, "Nate and I will back the line of credit completely. Every Sunday we will reimburse you for anything you sold on credit. We completely trust you to handle your customers with love and kindness. Please don't ever pressure anyone to pay. If someone is struggling, the four of us will develop a way for them to pay us back. You know we enjoy helping our neighbors." It was another good deed that Nate and Sharon provided for some members of the town; they loved helping. It didn't take long for Mary and Thomas to figure out the plan. They both were so proud.

Bethany was working a small amount of hours at the store the last few years. She was quite busy with family business – two little ones named Tom and Marybeth. The young father and mother could not believe the help that was constantly being offered. The entire Johnson clan plus Barbara wanted to help. Bethany had become a huge fan of Sharon and Mary. Both women helped in so many ways.

Lizzie was nineteen now and was engaged to Steve. They had been boyfriend and girlfriend for five years. Sharon and Nate really liked Steve. He was hard working, had some good skills, and adored Lizzie. He had passed Sharon and Nate's test last year with excellence. Lizzie was told to never tell anyone about the test. It was just a possible gauge on how much a man loves his fiancée. Miss Jacobs did tell Sharon that Steve passed with an A+. The test was something that Nate and Sharon had come up with right after Andy and Bethany's wedding.

After that regretful comment about Dr. Hemfield that disappointed his mother, Nate started thinking how terrible he felt. During his thoughts at the reception, he also thought about how he had disappointed Sharon. He couldn't believe the feeling he immediately experienced. It was terrible! He didn't know for sure, but he thought his chest hurt some. His brain started quickly filling with thoughts after the sensation. The idea of hurting, disappointing Sharon made Nate sadder than he had ever been in a long time, maybe his entire life. He never wanted to ever experience these things again. He didn't even want to think about it ever again. Nate was fully aware that the previous two men in Sharon's life did not treat her well. He wondered how could a woman really know whom to marry?

The next evening during their alone time, Nate shared his thoughts about how devastated he felt with the thought of disappointing the greatest wife and person that anyone could ever meet. Sharon hugged and kissed her husband for an extended time. She told him after the embrace that she felt very much the same way. During their ensuing conversation, they decided that a woman should ask their prospective husband if he would ever disappoint her. In the end, it was decided that Nate and Sharon would only explain this question-asking scenario about disappointment to their girls. It was quite detailed and had to be asked very discreetly. The timing of the question had to be perfect. Reading body language and facial expressions might provide the answer. Sharon told Nate that this question was a wonderful way to possibly find out how much a girl's fiancé loves her.

Steve and Elizabeth were so kind to Susie and Sally. The engaged couple was very busy with work, but they always took some time to interact with these new members of the family. Susie and Sally were doing extremely well in all endeavors. They were ten and thirteen now and handled their chores like experts. They both liked to work; they enjoyed doing things well. Two girls who had been so quiet and somewhat withdrawn had completely blossomed. They had been loved and supported by the entire Johnson clan; it showed. Sammy and Ruthie, who were best friends, did so much for the smallest workers at the JT. There were so many compliments and words of encouragement from these two that Susie and Sally responded by working harder to please everyone.

Nate and Sharon loved the interaction within the Johnson clan. Six senior mentors were wonderful. Dee and Mary taught cooking to Beth, Lizzie, and Ruthie, sometimes Sammy and Sharon would attend. It was always fun; Dee and Mary really enjoyed the interaction. Thomas and Nate taught so much about horses and cattle to Steve and Lizzie. Except for Nate's herd, Steve and Lizzie were taking over the cattle business. Sharon had taught both of them how to rope. Steve was a great cowboy and was very good in all aspects of the business. He was responsible for all sales, even the yearly sale of seventy-five head that ended up in Dodge City. Jeremy was teaching carpenter work to Sammy; they both really enjoyed their relationship. Sammy was always thankful for his kind mentor, and Jeremy enjoyed teaching about wood constructing.

Every day during the growing season, Nate and Sharon visited the garden. It was substantially larger than the one they started with eleven years ago. The Johnson clan needed it. There were now seventeen members enjoying the benefits of such a splendid garden. Everybody worked in the garden from time to time; it was considered family time.

Thomas and Dee mostly supervised, gave meaningful compliments to the workers, and were responsible for the very pleasant conversation. They were both sixty-six now; it was difficult for them to garden, but they loved being in the garden area, visiting, and enjoying the activity with the family.

Nate had an apprentice named Tom, a fifteen-year-old friend of Sammy's. It brought back memories for Nate of his time with Jack. He tried to be as good of a mentor as Jack was. Tom was a quick learner and was very appreciative of Nate's instruction. Sometimes they would help Jeremy and Sammy on certain wood projects. Nate always followed his father's lead. It brought back memories for both men, pleasant ones. Jeremy appreciated that his son, the owner of this wood shop, put him in charge. It showed what a kind and thoughtful man Nate was. Sammy and Tom really enjoyed working together. They would continue to do so for the rest of their lives.

The owners of the JT Ranch kept very busy during the day. Sometimes they taught separately. Their working together time wasn't what it used to be, so the couple loved working in the store together. Sharon thought being in the store was not work at all. She always arranged for Nate to be there. She has to see friends and be with the most important person in her life. Eleven years of marriage had not dimmed their love for each other. The kind words, compliments, and affection flowed between the married couple just as strongly as it did in the past.

Sharon's thoughtful husband had always written short letters and notes to her throughout their time together. Nate was following M's advice about written communication. Sharon loved the correspondence and read them repeatedly, but the one on their tenth anniversary was way beyond special.

Nate wrote a long letter in detail about some of his favorite times. He arranged the letter in three main parts. Sharon could not believe the longest section, by far, was the one about Nate watching HER do things or just plain watching HER. The next section was about things they had done together. She loved this one best of all. He mentioned in this section the ultimate bond that was created by being together and doing so many things as a couple. The highest level of love and affection that he felt for his rather amazing wife was reinforced every time he did things with her. Nate said the feeling is stronger now after ten years than it was in the first. The last section was about Nate watching Sharon interact with others. This part also mentioned the good deeds, kindness, and support she delivered to anyone she talked to. Nate explained near the end of the letter that watching her with others still warms his heart and brings him such joy. This is especially true when it comes to children.

Nate closed the letter with the fact that he loves supporting all the things his lovely wife does. He thought that Sharon had a gift with people. This allowed her to mentor and guide others to do great things. He closed the letter by telling Sharon, "Years ago you mentioned how special my mother and Marjorie were, the M and M2 team. I always thought M was beyond special, but you, my dear wife, have surpassed them both. You have the skills to teach so much, you have the love and kindness to compliment and support, and you live a life full of all the mannerisms that demonstrate friendliness and respect to all. You are touching so many lives in so many ways. I LOVE YOU SO, SO VERY MUCH."

Nate had so many memorable interactions with Sharon over the last ten years. One of his favorites was the day he told her that she was a puppy. He told her, "Everybody loves seeing and being around puppies; they give such joy. You are my puppy. You give me such joy, and I love being near you. I love seeing all the things you do." As he started to give Sharon a hug, he was concerned that she hadn't said a word. Maybe she didn't like his metaphor. As he initiated the hug, somewhat worried, Sharon quickly licked his cheek two times and said, "Ruff, ruff". Nate laughed and said that he loved her reaction to his words. He was sure he would smile every time he thought about his puppy. He did; who wouldn't.

One day while tending to Nate's herd, Sharon was talking about how large the Johnson clan had grown. She was impressed at how well everybody was doing. Nate stated, "I might be somewhat prejudiced, but I believe that working hard, being married, and living a kind and supportive lifestyle really benefit people. All three things enable folks to be happier. I really only need one though; can you guess?"

Sharon replied, "Well, you've always liked blacksmithing." She was smiling and had the twinkle in her eye that Nate loved so much.

He responded, "I'm going to tell mom."

They had heard those very words from Susan that morning when she and Sally were doing chores. They found out later that Sally had kicked Susan in the shin. Mary was there to handle the situation. Mary and Sharon disciplined in almost the exact same fashion. Both believed that mistakes were teaching moments. Sally was getting much better at controlling her temper, but there were lapses every occasionally.

Sharon rode Blackie over to Nate where he was "pushing" a few strays back towards the main group. She said that maybe they could hold hands for a minute to settle any differences of opinion. She was smiling and asked if her husband would please not tell mom. They did hold hands; Sharon squeezed her husband's hand three times.

Lizzie saw Nate and Sharon returning to the JT. She and Steve were outside getting four horses ready as they had rentals for an afternoon ride. Steve was taking them out. The renters were experienced riders; it would be an easy job for Steve. Sharon's old horse Rusty was now doing duty as a rental horse. He still liked to work, but he could not do the same moves he could when he was much younger. He was still Sharon's favorite. She just couldn't risk Rusty getting hurt. She handed Blackie off to Nate as she visited with her "old boy".

The owners of the JT went to work on their horses, brushing and then feeding those something special, peppermint rounds. Sharon had incorporated the treats shortly after the soldiers gave Nancy's and her horses the candy 11 years ago. Rusty was especially fond of them. He would get a couple later when Sharon visited him again. As the happy couple was brushing away, they heard wagons pulling up near the house. They both exited the barn where they saw Allen and Henry pulling two large wagons to a stop. One was the wagon from the previous visit four years ago. The other wagon did not appear to be connected to the orphanage. It looked just like the old wagon that the Moores had left behind when they went to California. In a short time, there were kids everywhere.

Mr. Avery approached, shook Nate's hand, said hello to Sharon, and apologized for just dropping in like this. He said that he was desperate. He explained that the orphanage where he and Henry work just burned down. They were able to temporarily house several children with local families, but there is no place for all the ones here.

Sharon took Nate's hand, squeezed it three times, and said, "It would be our pleasure to help. We have some fruit, freshly made cookies, and bread and meat for sandwiches. Are you hungry?" Nate squeezed Sharon's hand three times.

"We are all quite hungry. It has been a couple of rough days. Thank you for the lunch offer; we'll definitely take you up on your kindness. If I may, I do need to talk to you both about some pressing matters," said a smiling Mr. Avery. He noticed four people exiting the front door of the house.

The Johnson's three children along with Ruthie were approaching the group. They went right over to the twelve visiting children; Sally, Susan, and Sammy knew two of the visitors. All sixteen were engaged in conversation. Ruthie was doing most of the talking. She was laughing, smiling, and exhibiting some of the same mannerisms as Sharon. Mr. Avery was not surprised when he saw Sally and Susan doing the same thing. Sharon Johnson had that effect on people.

The children ate lunch as they walked around. They definitely did not want to sit down.

Ruthie and the three Johnsons showed them all the animals. Allen and Henry had a chance to talk to Nate and Sharon about the situation. The administrator explained once again that he had no place to put these children. He also had three more that needed placement back where they just came from. There is no money for food and other necessities. The orphanage has always depended on local donations for its survival. There is no place to live available in the town we just came from; there is nothing nearby. No one is going to build another home for the children. The church has always been very helpful, but it will now be too far away to help. He asked the Johnsons if they knew anybody who could help.

By this time, the children were coming back for any leftover cookies. Lizzie had made a rather large batch during lunch; she knew they would be very popular. She was not wrong. Mr. Avery suggested that the whole crew go on a hike up behind the house to see what is there. Ruthie stated that she would lead the way. Allen wanted to give Nate and Sharon some time to talk. He felt that they would definitely help some; he hoped for the best. He and Henry prayed for permanent residence for the entire group.

Sharon took Nate's hand as she started to talk. She explained that she had been somewhat nervous about the situation four years ago when adopting Sally, Susan, and Sammy, but the children needed help. At that particular moment, she remembered the lessons that M taught about the three stages of development. M2's lesson about children being the framework of a house also entered her mind. "I knew at that moment we could and should help these three children," said a watery-eyed Sharon.

She stopped talking and hugged her husband for a short time. Sharon thanked Nate for sharing those lessons. "I loved every second and every detail of those lessons, but the most important thing of all, more important than the children's needs, more important than the three stages of development or the framework lesson, was the fact that I had YOU there. We would work together. We would use your mentors' wonderful lessons and provide a loving and supportive home. We have done a wonderful job so far. I want to emphasize the word WE. I see the results every day." Sharon kissed Nate.

Nate held on to his wife as he said, "We have helped to build an amazing family. Four years ago, we had six senior mentors plus Lizzie and Andy. Now, we have added Bethany, Sammy, Steve, Ruthie, and Tommy. Susie and Sally are learning so much from everybody, but you are leading the way. The girls will start teaching things they have learned from their mentors. I have no doubt that the older orphanage children can also become mentors. I think helping children is what we are supposed to do. What do you think?"

"I don't think we have a choice. Our visitors have no money, no place to go. We have to let them stay here and at the boarding house. Even If we did have a choice, I would still say that they could stay here. The JT Ranch has provided us this opportunity to benefit others. I love what we do together; it completes me as a person. Thomas will be so proud," said a smiling Mrs. Johnson. Nate squeezed her hand three times.

When the "exploring crew" arrived back in the yard, Sharon told the group, "Nate and I have a plan to house everybody, including the three you left behind. The two adults and five oldest boys will be living at the boarding house. There are officer quarters for Henry and Allen, and the boys can bunk with the young bachelors who work in the area. They are all well behaved; Thomas has made sure of that. He owns the property. Poor behavior means no job, no place to live.

All the little ones will stay with us. Nate has just fired up the fire pit; there will be hot water in fifteen minutes." She explained how the shower system worked. Mr. Avery was very impressed. He had never had a shower before.

The oldest visitors started the showering process as the rest of the newcomers sat around the fire. Sammy and his little sisters entertained the little ones. Nate helped entertain, stoked the fire, and helped make the showering run smoothly. Sharon, Lizzie, and Ruthie started getting things ready inside the house. Henry and Allen, after their showers, were moving from place to place asking if they could help. Both men helped some, but they could not believe how the Johnson clan went right to work preparing everything. Everyone was smiling, making jokes, and talking during their preparations. There was no doubt who was leading the way. Nate started some campfire songs with Sammy providing the music. He had learned to play the guitar to impress Ruthie; he was quite good. Some of the kids were even dancing.

Allen started the showering process with a couple of the younger boys, and soon Sharon appeared on the scene to help the little girls. Ruthie helped them get dressed and fixed their hair. The little ones were quick to take a liking to both kind and caring women. Lizzie was continuing the dinner preparations. Nate and Sammy continued to entertain at the fire pit.

Dinner went exceptionally well; Nate really knew how to handle his fire pit. The meat and potatoes were tasty as was the salad and biscuits prepared predominantly by Lizzie. Steve came in towards the end of the preparation to help Lizzie. He asked Ruthie if she would take charge of caring for the horses. She had several offers from the visitors to help. Once again, the entire process impressed Allen. Nate and Sharon had created a clan of good workers; that is for sure. He was happy that a couple of the older boys had volunteered to help with the horses. Mr. and Mrs. Johnson had not even moved after all the showers were completed. They just continued visiting with the children at the fire pit... VERY TOUCHING

When all the family and guests were down for the night, Nate and Sharon had their nightly alone time. Sharon gave Nate a big hug and kiss. She told him, "Today was fantastic. Our family was so kind and supportive. You were unbelievably wonderful. Today I understood how incredibly proud Thomas feels about you. He and M helped mentor you into the man you are today. When he sees you and I do good things, it is as if Thomas is thinking 'look at what my creations are doing'. TODAY I SAW FIVE OF OUR YOUNGER JOHNSON CLAN MEMBERS DOING AMAZING THINGS. OUR MENTORING WAS ON DISPLAY TODAY. I LOVED EVERY MINUTE OF IT."

Nate was rubbing his wife's hand and arm as he told her, "I loved watching you today. You are so right; today was so special." He also said that he would always support her activities. "You made the perfect call today, but, more importantly, you made our visitors feel wanted. They will all grow into something special with you leading the way. I too was very pleased with our kids today. They will continue to do good things and be a positive support for others." They did indeed for many years to come.

Chapter 19

The Young Mentors

For the next ten years, Nate and Sharon participated in and watched a multitude of mentors being developed at the JT Ranch. The owners of the JT didn't have one particular job. They had become part time teachers and workers in a number of categories. Many days the two senior mentors worked together. Sharon didn't have anything to do with the cattle anymore. Eventually, Nate didn't work on projects with wood or iron anymore. Nate helped Sharon mentor roping and riding; she helped him teach about horses. Sometimes Nate would mentor in the wood shop or in the blacksmithing area. Sharon's domain was the garden; occasionally, Nate would watch. He still loved seeing Sharon interact with people.

The lessons taught by M and M2 were on display constantly. Nate and Sharon always complimented the workers. Their words, the smiles, and the positive heartfelt emotion provided the perfect support and motivation for everyone. The two mentors saw the results of their teaching often. There were wonderful compliments being given by many in the Johnson clan; smiles and positive support were everywhere. Mr. and Mrs. Johnson loved to see all the kindness and respect demonstrated by all. All the great things they were seeing energized Nate and Sharon. They, in turn, continued throughout the day to set the perfect example of being kind and doing positive things. They both knew that the little ones needed to see and hear these things many times to start to copy the behavior to some degree.

Nate and Sharon actually taught lessons together to the older "family" members. Their smile lesson was Nate's favorite. He and Sharon gave all the students a smile assignment just like M had done for her prized pupil. They had to report to the class in three days with a full report on how their smiles had affected the conversation. How did people react to the smiles? The Johnsons loved the discussion and input from all the students. In the end, Nate and Sharon were convinced that each student realized the power of a smile. Other lessons included topics like mistakes, oral communication, good deeds, positive influence, bullying, gossip, and work ethic. There were more; every lesson that Nate had written down in his journals was discussed. Sharon loved reading and talking about each lesson with her person. She knew the lessons as well as Nate.

Oral communication was a long involved lesson; it took many sessions. The couple did not want to rush this topic. They felt this lesson was so instrumental in delivering the knowledge a teenager would need to become a positive and supportive adult. M's words were always in Nate and Sharon's mind; "oral language is a beautiful tool that allows us to achieve so much, but oral language can do great damage. Beware"

Nate and Sharon explained that talking to others was the easiest way to deliver a message. I hope that it will always be uplifting. If the words need to be negative, tread lightly and try to be positive at the end of the talk. Negative words should be a rare occurrence. The couple talked about prying into someone's business, keeping opinions to a minimum unless asked to help, and joking around during competitions. These areas of conversation can lead to problems. It is best to be very careful during these times. As was the case in all their lessons, the Johnsons felt, in the end, the lesson was well learned. This was based on all the input from the students.

Nate and Sharon were fabulous together during the lessons. There were smiles and laughs; it was entertaining. Sharon was always the lead speaker; she was beyond great. Nate jumped in to add important parts or to enforce a point. His remarks were perfectly timed. Dan Perkins and Richard Jones attended a number of the lessons. Dan mentioned that he wished he had learned these lessons when he was a teenager. As a younger dad, he had said too many negative things to his son, did not compliment him enough, and dwelt on his son's mistakes for way too long. That is how he was raised. He thought that is what you were supposed to do as a parent. He now understood by looking around the JT that there was a much better way to interact with children. The old colonel agreed that these were wonderful lessons. He joked with Nate and Sharon that if they wrote the lessons down, he would publish them.

When Thomas was 68 years old, He decided that he would finance the building of a magnificent home for the boys at the JT Ranch. There was the perfect spot, not far from the JT house. The old vet wanted this project to be the culminating good deed by the Smiths. Because it was the last deed, it was going to be the most expensive and, by far, the best thing the Smiths ever built. This would be a perfect ending to a lifetime of giving. Thomas would talk with Nate and Sharon about the home. He definitely wanted their input on the design. Nate and Sharon were very happy about helping to design a home for the boys, and they were thrilled that Thomas and Dee were so excited about the project. It would really add to the beauty of the JT Ranch. It would also make everything easier for everybody at the ranch. All of the older boys traveled from the boarding house and back every day. The new home would be a real benefit. The older boys would spend the entire day and night at the JT. They would have more time to visit with the little ones; mentoring would definitely increase. This would be great for everyone. Thomas was thrilled with all the good things Nate and Sharon had done with the JT. The new home just might make it easier for them to continue to do good deeds and be a positive support. HE WAS SO PROUD.

Nate and Thomas agreed to have Barry Collins be in charge of the project. Jack and Mabel's sons, Henry and Donald, were coming over to help Barry build the home. They were young, but, like their dad, were very big and strong for their age. Barry had taken over from his dad. Barry was a great carpenter, and Jack was his best friend. It only made sense that Jack and his boys visited a number of Barry's job sites. Henry and Donald soon started working with Barry. After several years, the boys decided that carpenter work would be their profession. Jack was disappointed that the boys didn't pick blacksmithing as their livelihood but was happy that his friend was teaching the boys a worthy skill.

Barry hired some local workers to assist in the construction. Several boys from the JT Ranch were hired. Nate and Sharon thanked Barry several times for giving some "family" members a chance to learn something so valuable. The crew did such skillful work on the home that several other jobs in town quickly became available. It was very clear to many that it was only going to be a matter of time before Barry moved his business to where the jobs were. This created a situation for Jack and Mabel. They knew that their sons would want to move with Barry. They would have to say no to their boys or make the move as a family. One big plus to the move was the fact that the Browns would look forward to rekindling their bond to the Johnson clan.

The home was designed like a ranch house. The kitchen was an equal to the one at the JT house. The big room downstairs was spectacular. Nate, Sharon, and Barry did a marvelous job of sharing thoughts. The giant rock and wood fireplace dominated the room; people just stared at its magnificence. Eight large bedrooms upstairs and one downstairs topped off the perfect design. The three "architects" loved what they had designed. Nate and Sharon built the sign for the home. They named the structure, Sharon, Abigail, Marjorie, and Mary House – SAMM HOUSE for short.

One day Thomas took Nate on a buggy ride out to where the family always held their picnics. He told Nate that he couldn't walk up the hill anymore, but he had done so in the past. He had a big favor to ask. The kind old vet explained to his son, "There's two different levels on the hill. Both are small but quite pretty; one is a little higher than the other is. I would like to be buried there right next to M. I would like you and Sharon to be buried fifty years from now on the level right below us." He smiled when he said fifty. Nate understood the need for a smile.

Nate did smile; then said, "If I go first, do I get the top of the hill?"

Thomas laughed and thanked his former student for the humor. "This is always a touchy subject, but it needs to be discussed. I don't want it to be sad, so let's smile and laugh our way through the conversation." He went on to explain that it was his idea for M and him, your mother and father, and Jack and Mabel to be on the top tier. The second tier would be for all the direct offspring of three aforementioned couples. Down here in this beautiful area would be the rest of the Johnson clan, which could number into the hundreds over time. You know that I never do things in a rash manner, so could you have this place ready next week?"

"Absolutely," said a smiling Nate, "I have to build Lizzie a house first, and Sharon wants me to paint the SAMM House, but I think I can do it. Do you think two pieces of wood nailed together would do?"

Thomas laughed and told Nate, "I want to talk to Mary and Jeremy and will write a letter to Jack and Mabel explaining everything. I just feel that this is the final place M and I would like to be – overlooking you and Sharon. I know it will take some time making all the preparations. I will handle all the expenses. I would like my son and daughter to please design the upper two areas if you would."

"Dad, we would love to do that." Nate embraced Thomas briefly. They had been doing that on a regular basis for a while. It meant so much to each of them.

Four months earlier after talking to Dee and Nate, Sharon had an emotional interaction with Thomas. She told him, "You've done things for me better than anyone could have imagined. You have taught me more things than anyone could have imagined. We have shared smiles and laughs more than anyone could have imagined. You mean so much to me, more than I could have ever imagined. Can I hug you now?" They embraced for quite a while. Sharon had a few tears when she asked, "Would it be okay if I called you Dad occasionally?"

Thomas was quite emotional, but he managed to say, "Thank you for those words. I have loved you like a daughter for a long time. I would love you calling me Dad." He took Sharon's hand as they started back to the house. He held it the entire way and then kissed it when they reached the house. The next day Thomas was so happy; Nate and Sharon were now both calling him Dad. Nate had already talked to his father about calling Thomas Dad. Jeremy had always loved the fact that Nate had two moms. He thought having two dads was just as good. Jeremy knew Thomas loved Nate and had taught him so much over the years. It was definitely a name Thomas was entitled to. This title meant more to Thomas than words could describe.

A couple of days later, Nate and Sharon took a Sunday ride out to Thomas' family cemetery spot. They walked up the hill; Sharon had never walked to this location before. Nate knew that his wife really liked this spot; her facial expressions said it all. Sharon hugged Nate and apologized for her exuberance. It probably wasn't right to be so happy over a cemetery spot. She said that this is the most beautiful place on the entire ranch. She absolutely loved the terraced look. The six senior mentors overlooking their "flock". Mrs. Johnson spent the next five minutes explaining her design. Then she stopped, said she was sorry again, and asked Nate for his thoughts.

Nate took Sharon's hands, squeezed them three times, and said, "The vegetation, the rock formations, and a beautiful little pond in view from here make this location absolutely stunning. I understand why Thomas likes it so much. Your design, by the way, is fantastic. I love your creative genius."

Within a short time span after a family meeting, it was decided by the Johnson clan that the family cemetery would be the spot Thomas had chosen. The design was to be the one created by Sharon, and the name was to be "Legacy Park", thought of by Mary. In a short time, Jack and Mabel would be moving to town. They would bring all the wrought iron fencing that Jack had built around M. It was ample enough to fence in the entire upper area. It was Jack's best work. This speaks volumes of its quality. They would also bring Marjorie.

Allen and Henry couldn't believe the entire experience at the JT Ranch. Never in their life had they seen such success by the children. Sharon made a rule on a child's first day at the JT; the word orphan would never be used again. All of them were now family, members of the Johnson clan. Allen never sent a child to another home to be adopted the entire time the "houses" were being run at the JT.

He even traveled to the territorial government offices to explain the entire setting and support system that was being provided by the Johnson clan. He mentioned that the teaching and mentoring are superb. There is job training available or fully paid college if the child is so inclined. Food and clothing are never an issue. The Johnsons seem to relish the idea of spending virtually all their money on the children. The housing is better than the majority of the people in these great United States of America experience. He went on to explain everything about the two houses, the original JT Ranch house and the SAMM House. He even invited the chief administrator and his wife to come for a visit.

One of Henry's jobs was to take the younger children to school. He loved the interaction; he had learned to smile and compliment quite often. The kids really liked it. He also couldn't believe all the work that was being done at the JT. All the school-aged children had a chore or two before heading out to their lessons. Chores were done before breakfast. Nate, Sharon, Allen, and Henry helped supervise the chores. There were smiles and laughs abounding inside and outside the houses. There were many compliments given to the young workers. A crew of workers was preparing breakfast. Some of the older residents were already working on their daily jobs. First breakfast fed all the older children and the cooks, usually around twenty-one people. The cooks were paid employees of the JT; they normally ate as they cooked. Second breakfast was smaller but still numbered around sixteen.

The best customer at Beth's Store, by far, was the JT Ranch. Sharon told Andy that the JT didn't expect a big discount because of volume or family connection. It was she and Nate's desire to benefit the town with their purchases. The JT could afford to pay the going rate. The same was true at the town markets. All the "Johnson clan" from the JT Ranch had some money to spend. The children absolutely loved the town market and dance. Nate and Sharon didn't have anything to sell anymore, but some of the Johnson clan did. Nate and Sharon walked around visiting with their many friends. The Johnsons absolutely loved seeing their "children" dance and have a good time. The loving couple, the owners of the most profitable enterprise in the area, were, by far, the most popular people at the event. It brought back memories to Nate about how well liked Marjorie and Thomas had been at the farmer's market. WOW!

Dan Perkins and Rich Jones were doing well in their business ventures. They hoped to make enough to live comfortably for the rest of their lives. Dan never told Rich that he already had plenty of money, but he wanted to help his friend. The old colonel was thrilled with the income. He asked Dan one day if he thought there was enough money to donate to the JT. Both men had been honorary members of the Johnson clan for quite some time. It was just the way Sharon and Nate were. The two old friends both thought that the JT Ranch was doing so many good things. Dan surprised Rich when he said he was thinking about leaving his whole estate to the JT. Colonel Jones replied that he liked that idea. Rich added that the JT Ranch does amazing things for the town, and Nate and Sharon benefit and support every child they encounter... The Colonel had grown quite attached to all the children at the JT. The kids at the JT loved calling him Colonel; he liked it too.

Four years after Jack and Mabel moved to town, three of the older members of the Johnson clan had moved on to a better place. Dee was next to her first husband, Jeremy was high on his perch overlooking the beautiful view below, and Thomas was next to his beloved M. Nate and Sharon presided over all the services. They did a marvelous job, said some touching things, and celebrated, in words, what memorable lives these mentors of many lived. Nate designed the ceremony with Sharon doing most of the talking. He would step in at certain places. It was much like his parents at Marjorie's funeral. Jack and Mabel sang a few songs. Food and music at the JT provided the perfect endings to such special days.

Mary wanted only family to attend Jeremy's celebration of life. It was what Jeremy wanted. Thomas' event was a party with more than a hundred people in attendance. There was so much laughing, telling stories, and dancing; everybody enjoyed his celebration of life. These two men, one somewhat quiet and reserved, the other so talented with his words and smiles, had been great friends for almost 30 years.

Nate and Sharon turned their house over to Ruthie and Sammy after Jeremy's funeral.

Ruthie had dated two young men when she was in her teens. They were nice, but she told Sharon one day that she believed that her heart belonged to someone else. Ruthie's amazing mentor took her "daughter's" hands and said that it is important to follow your heart most of the time. Sharon asked if she might know this lucky young man.

Ruthie hugged her mom and said, "It's Sammy."

Of course, Sharon and Nate knew that these two were perfect for each other. They had watched the two over the years; the way they interacted was magical. They really valued each other; the smiles and laughs flowed very easily between the two. The young ones always enjoyed working together. Sammy had already told his mother that he loved Ruthie. Shortly after Ruthie's announcement to Sharon, the young couple married. They officially took over running the most important business at the JT – taking care of the children. The younger Johnsons lived with Nate and Sharon for a period. This was only natural. It was a great place for Ruthie and Sammy. Sammy grew up in the house and Ruthie loved everything about it. Nate and Sharon did tell the newlyweds that the house would be theirs in time. Ruthie wanted to name their new home, The JT House. Nate and Sharon thought it was a great idea.

Mary welcomed Nate and Sharon to the Small Ranch. Sharon had spent several nights with Mary after the funeral. Mary wanted the company; she had always been the talker in the family. She couldn't be alone; of course, Nate and Sharon already knew this. They kept the conversation, smiles, and laughs going strong. Every day the three would go to the JT to work and/or mentor. Mary slept in later than she used to, so Nate and Sharon cooked breakfast together. It was still so special for them.

A rather favorite time of the day for Mary was the one hour that she and G sewed together. M2 and G loved talking about so many things. The conversations reminded Mary of her talks with M. Who wouldn't love that? They thoroughly enjoyed creating clothes with different color combinations and designs. Mary was impressed with Sharon's creativity. Once a month Andy and family came for dinner. Bethany always joined the women to sew. She was a beginner, but Mary and Sharon enjoyed showing Beth the basics. With two little ones and a very active husband, the two elder Johnson women knew Beth would have to become proficient at sewing patches and mending tears. Nate and Andy kept the kids busy in the barn. Uncle Nate was special; he made things for the children, bought them little gifts, and was thoroughly entertaining.

Mary loved helping out with little Sharon. Ruthie was busy working at times, so the former teacher provided the helping hand. Mary taught some of the girls at the JT how to babysit; they loved it. She also taught many of the young women to sew, and Mary was often seen in the kitchen and, sometimes, in the garden. Teaching at the JT was so important to the senior female mentor. She did not teach school anymore. She let some of the younger college graduates handle that. Two of the college-educated helpers, the local minister and the town's main lawyer, were both former "residents" at the JT.

Nate still loved watching his Sharon in action; she was still so special. So many of M's lessons were on display, but what Nate really enjoyed thinking about were the lessons Sharon had taught him. They were not formal lessons; Mr. Johnson had just seen and heard them over time. His favorite one was his wife's attitude towards work. She put an equal value on all good work. It did not matter if it was mucking out the stalls, falling a tree, creating a fine piece of furniture, or delivering a baby. Sharon always used the words "good work" when thanking the individual. She might say something like "thank you for your good work; the JT will benefit because of what you have done". She always smiled and her words conveyed sincere appreciation. He figured out that this was why everybody worked so hard to please Mrs. Johnson.

Sharon also taught Nate something new about humor. After several years of marriage, T learned to use parts of funny past stories or jokes into a present day conversation. Nate and Sharon did this numerous times; it was so much fun. J even started a journal of funny stories with Sharon. They loved reading them together. Nate's favorite was "King Najo". It all started when Nate mentioned that he thought Najo would be a perfect boy's name for Lizzie and Steve's new baby, due in two weeks. (Na te Jo hnson)

J knew from his wife's facial expressions and the nodding of her head that she understood the humor. Sharon played along by saying that Najo is a royal name. It should be used only for, perhaps, a king. Nate agreed and gave his wife a hug. Two nights later after Susan and Sally had left; Nate appeared on the scene wearing a crudely constructed crown with the name King Najo on the front. Sharon quickly knelt down with her hands on the floor out in front of her. Her only words were, "My King that is a majestic crown." They were both laughing.

The amazingly matched couple laughed on and off about King Najo for years. Examples would be: King Najo asked Queen Sharon to have "a cherry" pie made for dinner. That night a sugar cookie with one cherry on top made its way to the table. The cherry was sprinkled with cookie dough. Nate tried to be serious, but he could not. After a quick laugh, he managed to tell the queen that it was exactly what he ordered. Another time Queen Sharon mentioned to her king that there were a few weeds in the garden. The next morning Sharon felt Nate getting out of bed; she just smiled. After breakfast, King Nao took his queen to the garden where ten rather large weeds had been added to the area that Sharon had cultivated yesterday. Sharon simply asked, "What did you say, my King, to your servant?"

He responded, "Weeds in the garden."

The Queen replied, "My King is so thoughtful. Every garden could use some more weeds."

After an amazing ten years, there were no longer any children living at the JT Ranch. There were three young women living at the JT House. They worked at the ranch. Sally and her husband lived in town, but Lizzie, Ruthie, and Susan, their husbands and children all lived at the JT. Brolins Construction had built Lizzie and Susan's houses. Brolins was a combination of Brown and Collins. Barry and Jack were still the best of friends and owned a highly successful construction company. Jack was the manager with Barry going back to what he loved, working with his hands. Both men had slowed down some, but both were very good with their workers. The owners had a plan for two of their best workers to take over the business. Both men were highly skilled. The owners of Brolins Construction knew them quite well; they were Donald and Henry.

All of the younger Johnson clan adults approached Nate and Sharon about making the JT Ranch a dude ranch after all the children left. They explained that the beautiful SAMM House was empty. Why not put it to use? There are so many things that people could do here at the ranch. Lizzie even mentioned that the lessons taught here to the children might be able to be continued. The group stated that they would handle everything. Nate and Sharon agreed to the plan. They both thought it might just be beneficial to many. They would also approach Allen and Henry about staying on at the JT in a different capacity.

Allen and Henry now helped run the dude ranch and supervised the activities at the boarding house. People could stay at the SAMM House, three cabins, or a well-done barracks. Ruthie and Sammy still ran the operation, but Henry and Allen were valuable assistants as there was much to coordinate. The guests at JT Ranch could choose from a variety of chores or classes. This is what made this place so special. People could work with wood or iron, ride and/or tend to the horses, work cattle, hike, or attend a class by Nate and Sharon to name a few. There were more options, depending on the season. It was still a working ranch. Some men wanted to fall a tree and/ or make lumber. Many women enjoyed the animals, making jam, and working in the garden and orchard. The classes were always the most popular items to choose from, and everybody who stayed at the JT Ranch always visited Legacy Park.

Nate and Sharon taught lessons from Nate's journals that the couple had discussed so often. Their favorite lessons, by far, were the ones about the power of a smile and the love of a spouse. Nate and Sharon taught M's words, but they also added some items they had discovered through the years. Most of the guests were young married couples who quickly became big fans of the Smiths and the Johnsons. Nate and Sharon did an amazing job with the classes. They missed the children they used to mentor, but these young couples were avid attendees. Every "student" left the classes a different person. Many couples exited the ranch with a better understanding about the love of a spouse. Marjorie's lessons, so loved by Nate and Sharon, were the main reason why many couples came to the SAMM House.

Ruthie and Sammy taught lessons on compliments and oral communication; they were quite good together. Ruthie was so much like Sharon. She even jumped up and down when she got excited about something; Sammy loved it. Sometimes they would take a group for a leisurely horse ride. Roping was also taught, but Sammy and Ruthie did these two things on a part time basis. Other staff members filled in when they were occupied elsewhere. Their primary job was running the dude ranch. They still loved working and being together. Nate and Sharon knew that this couple was going to be so happily married forever.

Allen and Henry loved talking to the guests about all the things that went on at the JT Ranch. They also liked reminiscing about all the "Johnson children" who had lived and prospered at the JT. They were both at the age where a person sometimes stops and reflects on what they had done during their lifetime. Both men felt proud and fulfilled by their accomplishments, especially their time at the JT Ranch. The SAMM and JT Houses had closed as an orphanage because of the growth of churches, much larger towns, and a very improved standard of living by so many in the area. The local community now handled most orphans, but many senior members of the clergy up to 200 miles away were very aware of the gold standard of orphanages, The JT Ranch.

Nate tried to get Legacy Park ready in time for everybody, but he fell short of his goal. Nate and Sharon had spent many days at Dan Perkins' old mine site. They loved riding over and collecting rocks for the walkway up the hill at Legacy Park. Nate and Sharon timed it so that all five direct descendants of the upper tier mentors and their families would finish the walkway up to and inside the upper tier of Legacy Park. Nate had spent weeks preparing the pathway and the spots for the headstones. It was slow work, but Nate wanted it to be perfect. He had seen many slanted headstones. Nate wasn't going to have that happen.

Jack, Mabel, and Mary sat and watched as their families carefully placed each rock.

After several hours, an enjoyable lunch was served. Nate and Sharon had prepared the picnic lunch. Sharon mentioned to Mary while eating that they were sorry they hadn't gotten everything done in time for Jeremy's service. Mary told her son and Sharon that when she is here at this stunning location, there is absolutely no room for a negative thought. The design and the workmanship are magnificent, so, please, never another negative word about Legacy Park.

Over the years, the Johnson clan gatherings at the JT changed significantly. There were often ten married couples with many children running around. Mac and Doris had the oldest ones on the scene. With train service being so close now, the Jones family made frequent visits to the JT. Their children loved the ranch. Some of the older children had a word they used occasionally, "Sharon like". When one of the many young folks did something very nice, someone in the group might say, "That was very Sharon like." It was meant as the highest compliment possible. Nate loved it.

Doris and Mac always visited Legacy Park when they came to the ranch. They were so impressed with everything; everybody was. Nate had been in charge of designing the headstones; Mary and he wrote the first three. Nate wanted to give Marjorie a much larger headstone, one that mentioned more about her amazing life. He felt that Thomas was unable to correctly mention the proper words because of his condition. He still had been so overwhelmed when he created the first headstone. Nate told his mother that he meant no disrespect. She agreed 100%. All three headstones were of the same design. Each one had five sections: a wide sculpted base, three sections where the words were written, and a wonderfully designed top piece. Each piece could be moved up the hill individually and then put together. Nate's idea for a wide solid base for each stone to keep them from leaning away from vertical seemed to work beautifully. People commented on the beauty of the headstones and the words inscribed on them.

Nate and Sharon had built a rather large sign just to the left of the gate where you entered the upper tier. Mary said she loved the words and the way they were delivered.

THESE SIX PEOPLE

AMAZING IN SO MANY WAYS

THEY ALL SMILED OFTEN; THEY KNEW THE POWER OF A SMILE

THEY WERE KIND TO ALL; KINDNESS MAKES EVERYBODY BETTER

THEY GAVE GREAT COMPLIMENTS TO MANY, ESPECIALLY KIDS

THEY KNEW COMPLIMENTS MOTIVATED PEOPLE TO BE BETTER

THEY HELPED; HELPING PROMOTES SMILES AND KINDNESS

THEY WERE POSITIVE AND SUPPORTIVE TO ALL PEOPLE

THEY KNEW THESE THINGS HELP BUILD STRONG FAMILIES

ALL SIX DEMONSTRATED TO ALL

THEY ARE EACH DESERVING OF THE SPECIAL WORDS

A LIFE WELL LIVED

Chapter 20
the Waning Years

Legacy Park was pretty much completed. Nate and Sharon decided to get help in finishing all three sections. Nate had felt terrible about not getting the top tier ready in time for the first two services. He didn't want that to happen again. Tommy and his apprentices did all the wrought iron work. Other workers at the JT collected all the rocks, and the family secured the ground under each headstone area. Right after Thomas' service, Sharon mentioned to Nate about the possibility of placing Dan Perkins and Colonel Jones up on the hill. It was her intention to keep Nate busy with conversation and work until he was able to get back to normal. He had taken Thomas' passing hard. Sharon struggled also, but her focus was taking care of Nate. She used the same techniques that were used on her many years earlier. She had never forgotten what Nate did for her.

Nate thought it was a splendid idea. He and Sharon traveled out to Legacy Park to check out the spot his lovely wife had mentioned. Mrs. Johnson kept her husband busy with conversation the whole time. She held his hand often and gave him several hugs. It was decided that these two men had been instrumental in making this town such a wonderful place to live. Dan started everything by inviting Thomas to come for a visit. He was the one who convinced Dr. Smith to move. Colonel Jones agreed to build the outpost and provide security. Both things were critical in moving the town forward. The spot was off to the side and slightly behind the upper tier. Nate liked the spot. The walkway was almost done, and the area looked like it was going to be easy to prepare.

Nate arranged for the two men to meet him and Sharon at Legacy Park while on their way to their lumber mill. Sharon would do all the talking. Nate knew the men couldn't say no to her, very few could. The Colonel walked up the hill with the Johnsons while Dan sat in the buggy. When Sharon pointed out the spot, Rich thought it was stunning. He said, "I really don't have a burial spot planned out, probably just a military cemetery way off in the distance. I feel a strong connection to this town. I will always be indebted to you and Nate for allowing me to be a member of the Johnson clan. This family and my military career are the highlights of my life. This is a real honor. Thank you." He stopped as he was tearing up.

Sharon smiled and suggested a snack as they walked down. Colonel Jones loved the idea of a snack while visiting with the Johnsons; they were so pleasant to talk to. The three stopped several times to enjoy the view. Upon reaching the buggy, Rich explained to Dan what he saw up on the hill as he continued to munch on one of Sharon's biscuits and jam. Dan agreed to the plan wholeheartedly after his friend described the spot. During the friendly conversation, Nate mentioned that his sister was a very good writer. She is writing a short history of this town during all the years the Johnsons have been here. The pamphlet stops with Thomas' internment. Both of you two men are mentioned often.

Dan chipped in with, "Sign me up for a hundred copies. I will give them to everyone I know. I've always wanted to be famous." He was smiling.

Rich pointed out to his friend that he was already famous; Dan owns the best mine in town. Everyone laughed as Dan sarcastically stated that it has made him famously rich.

Nate quickly added, "You've known Rich for a long time then."

Dan ended the joking by saying, "I like spreading my wealth around. You three walked up Legacy Park on some of my wealth."

Sharon took Dan's hand with both of hers and told him that the rocks really enhance the beauty of this place. She thanked him for letting the family have them. The walkways are perfect. The old lawyer responded that being part of something so beautiful is an honor. Thank you both so much for this amazing gesture; you are so kind.

As the Colonel was entering the buggy to continue out the road to their lumber mill, he told Nate and Sharon that he just needed one copy of Doris' pamphlet. He was going to send it to the Smithsonian in Washington. Everybody laughed.

Sharon explained to the men, "That's only fitting. You did know that the building is named after Dr. Thomas Smith, right?" more laughs

As Dan and Rich continued out to the mill, the lawyer mentioned to his friend, "It's so easy to leave my estate to these two wonderful people. The paperwork is all done. Nate and Sharon never stop thinking of other people. They are paying for a college tuition for one of their 'kids' who lived at the JT. One more is going to college soon. How great is that? They mentor everybody at the ranch and beyond. I can't think of a single person in town who doesn't admire the work they do. John Jacobs runs the Johnson wood mill; he does an excellent job. He is also a fine mentor to his younger staff even though he is, by nature, a quiet man. One day the topic of Nate and Sharon came up as we were visiting. I couldn't believe how John went on and on about Nate and Sharon. He basically said that the Johnsons make everybody better. He loves watching them interact with people. His girls and he love them dearly for who they are and what they have done for them and so many others. My estate couldn't be in any better hands."

Colonel Jones agreed that Nate and Sharon were more than special. He stated, "I am pretty confident that my estate will go to the same place, unless of course, I get married in the next few years." Dan laughed as he thought about how much his friend was making jokes and smiling when talking to others. He hadn't been that way as a soldier. Dan knew his friend learned these things from Sharon and Nate. He told Rich that any woman would be lucky to have such a dashingly good-looking soldier who could lead a cavalry charge with the best of them.

The Colonel countered with the fact, "My old horse can't travel any faster than a light canter. I would do a great job in slow motion." "Kinda like I walk," quipped the old lawyer.

Sharon was hit hard by M2's passing, harder than Nate was. Mary had been so kind and loving to her. Sharon had grown quite close to Michelle Moore, but that friendship was only one and a half years long. Sharon had known M2 for about 22 years. During that time, the two developed a relationship much like Marjorie and Mary. The younger Mrs. Johnson learned so much from Nate's mother. M2 was always a joy to talk to; she was funny, a wonderful listener, and very personable. Sharon had really liked sewing with M2.

Nate quickly sensed his wife's sorrow. This is why he asked Sharon if Mabel could move in for a short time. Mabel had lost Jack six months earlier. Sharon said that she would like that for a short time. Mabel was living with Donald and his family. Henry was close by with his family. The living quarters at Donald's weren't wonderful. Mabel did indeed want to help Nate and Sharon; she adored both of them. They also had a rather large bedroom available; that would be nice. Donald was going to build an addition onto his house for his mother, but it couldn't happen until spring.

Mabel sewed with Sharon every night. They visited about so many things. Sharon loved hearing stories about when Mabel became a member of the Smith family and later, the Johnson clan. They too loved designing different color and style combinations of clothes. It brought back memories of Sharon's sewing with Mary. Sharon had learned so much from M2. She taught Mabel so much in a short time that their products were appearing in Mary's Clothing Store. Andy had opened Mary's Clothing Store after Sharon and his mom started to accumulate finished products. They were making some very nice dresses and blouses. Andy figured there was a need for a place to sell the merchandise. Several young women who Mary had mentored in sewing also contributed to the store. There was also fabric for sale. Mary had really liked the store; she was often seen there. She gave sewing tips to many. She liked that. She had never gotten tired of teaching.

Nate was a real benefit to his wife during this time. Mabel was brought in to assist, but Nate accompanied Sharon every day at the JT. They no longer worked separately. They held hands and continued to mentor, compliment, and bring smiles everywhere they went. Sharon enjoyed working as a team. They continued this style for the rest of their lives. In time, Nate held up Sharon's right side when they walked together. He was still very strong and loved helping. Even though she depended on her husband's strong left arm, it didn't stop her from demonstrating all the mannerisms that made her so well loved. Sharon's physical early years had somewhat caught up with her, but she never complained.

Mabel did move out in the spring. She and Sharon had grown so much closer. Some days Mrs. Johnson would pick up Mabel at Donald's and they would work at Mary's Clothing Store and/or the Town Store until early afternoon. After a lunch with a wonderful friendship being demonstrated between the two, Sharon would drop Mabel back off at Donald's house where she would help babysit. Sharon would ride out to the JT where she would meet up with her person. Each missed each other during the morning. Nate mentioned that he knew what she was doing in town was very worthwhile, but his hand was missing its partner. He quickly kissed her on the cheek and said being apart makes the afternoon and evening even more special than normal. He squeezed her hand three times.

On most nights Sharon sewed by herself, but she did have a very likable attentive attendant. Nate rubbed her feet, brushed her hair, and massaged her right knee.

Sometimes she would take a break, and he would rub her back. He absolutely loved doing these things for his Sharon. Every night he would incorporate a few comments about sunshine. Nate had made his wife a beautiful plague that hung over the door that said "YOU ARE MY SUNSHINE".

Sometimes one or two of the girls would come over to sew; it was usually two. Lizzie and Ruthie came together as did Sally and Susan. Sharon loved telling Nate a day or two before that our girls are coming over to sew. Nate would usually visit for a few minutes and then excuse himself. He would work in the barn for a couple of hours. The girls always went out to the barn to say good night. Their entire families loved him so very much. He was such a gifted mentor and role model. His kindness to others was visible everywhere he went. Everyone saw how he treated his amazing wife. Nate was always supporting, complementing, and helping Sharon in all ways possible. He was so kind to give them their "girl time".

Of course, Nate and Sharon always enjoyed their evening talk after the girls left. Sharon would update Nate on everybody. He enjoyed hearing about the grandchildren. As was their custom, they discussed the day; the laughs, the joys, and the wonderful interaction at the JT. The staff at the JT Ranch provided living examples of Nate and Sharon's lessons. All the guests visiting the dude ranch saw this and were interested as to why the staff was so happy. This motivated many to want to learn more about the lessons posted on the board on the porch. The elder Johnsons never tired of seeing the quests "living" M's lessons. Nate was so happy that he had given Doris his journals from many years ago.

The last thing the couple did every night was pray. Sharon always spoke while holding hands with Nate. Over the many years of nightly prayers, Nate noticed that Sharon very seldom asked for anything. She, instead, thanked the Lord for keeping the family healthy and safe that day. She always thanked Him for allowing the family to give to others. She would often give details on which family members gave. Nate loved listening to his wife pray. He didn't know if there was such a thing as good prayers or not, but T was special. It was as if she was talking to a friend.

The Johnsons had always taught Thomas' lesson about the power of giving to each resident of the JT individually. The couple still mentioned the lesson to guests on an individual basis if it happened to be appropriate to the conversation. They felt by doing the lesson in this manner there would be no pressure about giving. People shouldn't be pressured to give. Nate and Sharon loved the multiplier effect of giving. It was always explained in a story Sharon shared with the student. Sharon mentioned that a young man who had no material things to give often helped a nearby family do things around their place. They really needed the help, and he had the muscles and the desire to assist. Over a period of time, Sharon noticed that all four members of the family the young man was helping were, in turn, helping others. The young man was so proud that his giving was being passed on. In addition, yes, the giving continued to spread throughout the town. SO AMAZING TO SEE

Nate and Sharon decided to add to Thomas' lesson on giving. Sharon suggested that giving of your time was so positive and neighborly. Nate concurred wholeheartedly and added that he also had something that might fit. The happily married couple had been talking during breakfast about the town softball game the day before. They used to play, but, nowadays, they just cheer everyone on. Nate thought it would be cute to see if he could use a softball analogy. Nate said to his wife, "Let me throw something at you and see if you "catch" it." Sharon jumped up and assumed a catcher's position.

She quickly signaled for a fastball, put her hands out in front of her, and yelled out, "Give me your best fastball."

Nate got into his best pitching stance; he tried not to laugh, but he did. He did manage to blurt out, "Abigail reviewed lessons with M, M reviewed lessons with me, and I think we should review kindness, respect, smiles, and compliments when we teach about giving. Giving these things to people makes everyone and everything better. They should be mentioned often." Nate did a double windup to let Sharon know the pitch was coming. He showed the small apple that had been in his pocket and released the pitch underhanded.

Sharon caught the apple, threw it at a raven who was near the garden, and yelled out, "He was trying to steal." Nate laughed and then told his wife while smiling that she was the best catcher in the family. No raven was going to steal on her. He would add "the catcher" to his journal collection of funny interactions with his wife.

Nate and Sharon were celebrities at the JT Ranch. Their presentations were always noteworthy. The Johnsons displayed all the lessons they had learned so long ago as they taught these older "students". The guests enjoyed the humor, smiles, respect, compliments, and so much more. Nate and Sharon never rushed off after a lesson. They visited and answered questions for long periods. There were a number of guests who had read Doris' pamphlet about the history of the Johnson family and several others about M's lessons. All of these generated questions. Luckily, Nate and Sharon had helped Sammy build a couple of high chairs; they were very comfortable. They gave lessons from the chairs and answered many questions from the same spot. Sharon's knee "thanked" Nate for the idea of the high chairs.

Ruthie told Sammy one night that she thought some of the returning guests actually came back to learn more from Nate and Sharon. She mentioned that she thought this was the supreme acknowledgement of mentoring well done. She was able to see this first hand a short time later. A young couple checked into the SAMM House. They were walk-ins. Most people reserved rooms beforehand; modern conveniences like phones allowed this. This couple wanted to stay just two nights and paid in advance, somewhat unusual. Ruthie asked them what their plans were while staying at the JT Ranch. The couple replied that they just wanted to look around and maybe meet Nate and Sharon Johnson.

The chief administrator of the ranch had never heard that request before. People usually came to ride, work, and maybe attend some classes. Ruthie was very surprised when the couple asked about a small ranch nearby. As she was finishing checking them in, she mentioned that Nate and Sharon Johnson were on the premises. She would be glad to introduce them. The three walked over to the JT House where Nate and Sharon were visiting with Sammy and Tommy. As the two men excused themselves to go back to work, the senior Johnsons turned and saw Ruthie approaching with two strangers.

When Sharon saw them, she asked the man "Is your last name Moore?"

The young man smiled, but before he could say anything Ruthie asked her mom, "How did you know that? You're right; this is Thomas Moore and Michelle Moore."

By now, Nate realized what was going on; he had a big smile on his face. Sharon's facial expressions said it all; she had the biggest smile. Her eyes watered up in her excitement. Nate knew that this was a very special visit. Sharon had mentioned the Moores several times over the years. Nate knew that she had missed her best friend for quite a while. They both would enjoy hearing about the Moore family.

"Are you the grandchildren of Tom and Michelle Moore?" Sharon asked.

Thomas replied, "Yes we are; Wyatt is our dad. We both go to the University of

Oklahoma in Norman. We have wanted to visit for a couple of years now; today we did. By the way, Thomas and Michelle are our middle names; please call us Nate and Sharon."

Sharon had a few tears rolling down her cheeks, Nate's eyes were watered up, and Ruthie stood there, utterly amazed. Sammy got the full report later that day. They too liked to share their day with each other every night. Nate and Sharon took the guests on a short walk and then to the porch where they all sat and visited. From what Ruthie overheard during the conversation on the porch, these two guests had learned many lessons from their parents. The lessons were fully implemented into their lifestyle. Some of these lessons were from Sharon who had shared them with Michelle during their many hours of being together. UNBELIEVABLE

The Johnsons and Moores spent the entire afternoon and dinner visiting about their families. It was wonderful to find out that Tom and Michelle had been so happy for all these years. Mr. Moore had found a good paying job. He became one of the bosses after several years. Michelle fell in love with all the wonderful colors that were so popular in Mexican culture. She owned three clothing stores and, according to her grandkids, made a lot of money.

The elder Johnsons had taken their visitors out to the sawmill right after meeting them. They showed the young Moores the plague that was hung there by their grandfather about thirty years ago. Nate always took care of the sign over the years. It was and always will be very special to the owners of the JT. Both of the Moores were very emotional. This plague was part of their family's history. The words on the sign exemplify what Nate and Sharon had done for the Moore family. The young Moores knew the complete history of their family's time at the JT Ranch, and this was why they were so emotional.

The next morning the elderly Johnsons took the Moores on a tour of the Small Ranch and then out to Legacy Park. The Moores were absolutely in no rush. They took their time looking around, asked many questions, and explained how much they had heard about this place. When they arrived at Legacy Park, young Nate asked Sharon if this was the place where she had put on a roping and shooting display. Sharon simply said that it was. She hadn't ever talked about it, not even to Nate. She had only done it to prove a point. Sharon had never felt completely good about what she had done. Young Nate smiled as he said that his dad still talks about the best "cowboy" he is ever seen. Young Sharon added that our grandmother taught many of the lessons she learned here to a number of people who worked for her.

The Moores walked up Legacy Park; they read every headstone. Nate and Sharon did not walk up the hill. Sharon said no to the trip up the hill, so Nate sat next to her and held her hand. He told the love of his life that the Moores and Johnsons could each use some alone time. He squeezed her hand three times. Young Sharon asked about Dan Perkins and Colonel Jones when she and her brother came down. Nate explained they were considered family. Both of the Moores were excited about how stunning the park was. They loved the way the park was designed. They guessed that the middle level was empty because it is going to hold the descendants of those on the top tier. That is so very touching. Nate Moore said that he couldn't wait to tell his family about Legacy Park. The Moores then asked about the headstones they had seen in the barn at Small Ranch. Nate explained to the visitors, "I wanted to write Sharon's headstone because I am her biggest fan by far. She's too modest to explain her legacy."

Sharon simply said, "Nate is my rock, my foundation; everything I am built from him." She hadn't wanted to say anything. Normally, she would have hugged her husband and given him a kiss after such touching words, but she thought that might be inappropriate.

She still wondered how her Nate could love her so much. WHAT A BLESSING

That night Nate mentioned to Sharon, "Some people might think we are somewhat like celebrities, but I don't feel that way. We have just taught our family the lessons that we learned. I love the kind of people we have raised. You deserve most of the credit. I thoroughly loved being beside you during the entire journey. We should be proud of what we have done. Our good deeds are almost too many to be counted. Thomas was so right when he said that we would do great things together."

Sharon added, "I am so proud of the work we did with the Moores. We took in total strangers, helped them when they needed it the most, and taught them a few things along the way. I will enjoy thinking about them often from here out; it makes me so happy to do so. I also think about Abigail's lesson about a life well lived and how to achieve it. I think we qualify. To accomplish something as profound as taught by the most amazing person, Marjorie Smith is very special. We have experienced a life well lived. Words can't describe my feelings for you right now." She kissed him three times.

The next morning Nate and Sharon shared breakfast at the SAMM House with the

Moores. Ruthie, Lizzie, Susan, and Sally prepared breakfast and then joined the four for the meal. Other guests were at another table some distance away. They were one large group, a family reunion. Nate Moore asked if Sharon had a short lesson, she might share during breakfast. Mrs. Johnson nodded her head while displaying that wonderful smile. She also had a twinkle in her eye. She explained the lesson is called "everyone a flower", and Sharon was going to have the girls explain it.

"A couple of years ago when Mom was a teenager," said a smiling Ruthie, "a kind elderly gentleman taught my mom this lesson. He said that he treats every person he meets like a flower. All flowers bring some degree of beauty. They are appreciated, very worthwhile, and should be valued. Even a prickly cactus blooms wonderful flowers. The man continued to say that when he meets someone, his mind pretends they are a flower. He subsequently sees the beauty and value in them. He appreciates the time they spend with him and any worthwhile conversation they share. He always shows the utmost respect and smiles as much as he possibly can. In almost all his visits with folks, he gets the smile and respect back. Isn't that great?"

Sally mentioned that her mom practiced these things so much they became a permanent part of her interactions with others. Susan added that as a young man the kind elderly man saw so much violence: fights, shootings, slaps, and punches. Most of these things started with ugly words. Occasionally, the young man had used ugly words himself. He knew these ugly words coming from his mouth would have to be completely stopped. That is when he decided he would think of people as a flower; he loved the beauty of flowers. He would only use words that might get the other person to "bloom". He equated a smile to a bloom. His words worked most of the time.

Sharon Moore spoke, "We want to thank you all for this wonderful lesson. I believe we will use this lesson all the time; it is so easy to remember. It has such great results. It has some aspects of Marjorie's lesson on oral language, but it is somewhat more precise. It is very easy to implement in any conversation. We definitely think it will benefit everyone we visit with. I like the idea of thinking of people as a flower and trying to get them to bloom. Sharon, thank you so much for bringing this lesson to the JT Ranch; I would bet it is very popular.

"This has been one fantastic visit; one that we'll never forget. It will be a topic of conversation for years to come. Thank you all for being so kind. Nate and Sharon, you are everything my family says you are. Thank you for all the time you shared with us and all the pleasant conversation about this place and your family. We will proudly carry your names with us as we travel through life, attempting to emulate your good deeds and wonderful words."

The goodbyes between the groups were touching. The Moores told the girls that it was such a pleasure to meet them and their families. The younger residents of the JT and Sally thanked the Moores for coming to the ranch. They added that it was a joy meeting them. It would be fantastic if they could visit again. The goodbye between the Nates and Sharons was quite emotional. Both women cried some, and the men's eyes watered up. The words spoken by the Moores were words that would stay attached to the Johnsons' hearts for the rest of their lives.

Ruthie took the Moores to the train depot. The depot was just past Dan Perkin's old mine land. On the ride, Ruthie explained a few more things. The Moores really enjoyed being informed by Ruthie that many members of the family use the word Sharon like when complimenting someone who had done something very kind or supportive. It is a very special word, loved by everybody, but not used in Sharon's presence. It might embarrass her. Ruthie also mentioned that in the last five years Nate and Sharon have started using the words "wonderfulness" and "positivity". They both love the sound of those words. They enjoy using the two words occasionally in their conversations.

Sharon said, "This visit has been one of the highlights of our lives. We will definitely explain the word Sharon like to our grandmother; she will love it. I really like Nate and Sharon's new words. My brother and I are going to teach school. I can see us using those words often in class. I also enjoy the sound of each." Both of the Moores thanked Ruthie with a big kiss on the cheek to go along with a giant hug when they departed the buggy at the depot. These friends did stay in contact for many years to come.

At breakfast earlier in the day, Mrs. Sharon Johnson told the Moores that their entire clan has been and always will be connected to the Johnson family. They were all welcome to visit anytime; it would be such great fun. Sharon and Nate Moore did correspond with their namesakes for a number of years. The Moores' letters were long and very detailed about everybody in their family; the Johnsons loved every word. The owners of the JT replied to each letter, writing it together. Michelle would write occasionally. Sharon thoroughly enjoyed the correspondence from her previous best friend. She would always write something very special to her first sewing instructor.

One day while Nate and Sharon were sitting and talking on the porch at the Small Ranch, Hank English and his right-hand man, Rob Talbert, pulled up. Sharon had known Hank for about 45 years. Hank never married and was known as a very good and talented worker. He was somewhat of a quiet man; living alone, many times, promotes that particular personality trait. Nate knew Hank some; both respected each other for the good work they produced. As long as the Johnsons could remember, Hank English had never missed a town council meeting at the town square. He was a polite man who very seldom shared his opinions with others, but Sharon thought he enjoyed listening to people's thoughts. Nate and Sharon figured Hank came to the meetings just to see people and say his greetings to a few acquaintances. Most people like to visit some. The one person Hank seemed to enjoy was Sharon.

Rob apologized for intruding but said he made Hank come. "Don't shoot him; I'll take the blame." He smiled.

Sharon stood up and said, "I was just going to get my rifle. Now I know who to shoot." She smiled and shot a wink at the two visitors.

Nate was also smiling as he stood and stated, "Don't run off. Let me get you some tea. It would be the neighborly thing to do; then Sharon can shoot you."

Hank joined in, "Thank you three for the laughs. Rob makes me smile and laugh often. Isn't that great? He does most of the work at the ranch and makes all the decisions. My grown-up apprentice is such a blessing. After Rob and Jenny get married next month, they will become the owners of my ranch."

As Nate smiled and nodded, Sharon exclaimed, "How marvelous for everybody!"

Rob remarked, "Hank has taught me so much, and now he's giving Jenny and me his ranch. We are truly blessed to know this kind and wonderful man."

Hank thanked Rob for his words and said to Nate and Sharon, "My right-hand man brought me out here to give you a sign. Well, actually, he convinced me to give you the gift this morning. He loaded it and drove me out here, knowing full well that he might get shot."

He smiled. "I just kind of came along for the ride."

As the four walked to the back of the wagon, Rob told the Johnsons that Hank made this sign years ago. When the young man revealed the sign, Nate was amazed at the workmanship and Sharon could not hold back the tears.

OUR CHILDREN

ARE AN IMPORTANT PART OF

OUR LEGACY

Sharon hugged Hank and whispered, "Nate and I have made a number of signs. This one is the most beautiful and the words are truly fantastic. This sign in the town square is perfect."

Over the years, the time Nate and Sharon spent at the JT dwindled. They spent more time doing a few chores at their place and writing letters to their clan. They loved the entire bunch, not just the locals. Both Johnsons had shared their thoughts with family on how "flowers "disperse throughout the land. They spent some time every day in their garden that now included flowers. There was no need for a large productive garden like in the past. The garden at the JT was huge; everybody worked in it. The time in the garden was still a family event. There was laughing, wonderful conversation, and so many compliments. Sharon led the wonderfulness of the occasion from her old high chair. Nate worked in both gardens but really focused on the little one at the Small Ranch. Sharon would sit in her chair telling him what a good job he was doing as she led a conversation that contained so many memories. Nate loved it. The positivity of the conversation gave the old married couple such joy.

It was during this enjoyable activity that the couple decided to make a small sign next to the entrance to the second tier of Legacy Park. All family members who were to be at this level agreed to the sign. Nate and Sharon thoroughly enjoyed working together on the project. It brought back some very pleasant memories. They both thought the new sign was an integral part of the JT Ranch.

THE JOHNSON CLAN CHOSE TO FOLLOW A LIFE PATH

CREATED BY GOD. HIS TEACHINGS OF KINDNESS

AND GIVING WERE DEMONSTRATED IN SO MANY

WAYS. THE FAMILY IS VERY PROUD THAT THIS IS PART

OF THEIR HISTORY.

The couple still enjoyed cooking together. This amazing pair still loved each other's company so much. The conversation was not quite as exciting as they cooked nowadays compared to their "young love" days, but the dialogue was more meaningful. There were days when Nate and Sharon didn't even leave the Small Ranch. The entire family understood. Sharon's new joke was how "knowledgeable" Nate's hands were. She was always telling Nate that his "smart" hands could do so much. He was doing most of the work. He loved every minute of it because his Sharon was next to him. Nate would always help his wife as they walked around the ranch. At night his hands knew exactly how and where to rub her achy joints. He still was fueled by his wife's smile and kind words. Whenever possible, they kept cut flowers in the house.

The senior members of the Johnson clan loved their time at the JT. They would generally sit on the porch while visiting and watching the interaction between the families. Lizzie and Steve were grandparents. Sharon loved taking Nate's hand, squeezing it three times, and telling him that he was a great grandpa. The patriarch of this family never got tired of hearing this; it was so special to him. Nate always felt that Thomas had been the patriarch of the Johnson clan here in this town. He was the one responsible for Nate and Sharon being married with children. Dr. Smith had purchased the JT Ranch, a place that benefited family, friends, and so many children.

As Nate sat there holding his wife's hand while looking at the people and the land, he knew what it felt like to be the leader of this clan. The patriarch still had a very sharp mind. He was fully aware that he was holding the hand of the true "architect" of the building of this incredible family and wonderful ranch. Sharon had been the primary factor in making sure that every child felt wanted and, more importantly, was a member of the Johnson clan. Some children had no official family name upon their arrival. The owners of the JT Ranch always, at the right time, asked if they wanted to be adopted. There was never a negative response. Nate and Sharon were proud parents of eight children.

That night as Nate lay in bed with Sharon asleep with her head on his chest, he thought of his mother's words from years ago. She had said, "Thomas told me that you were he and Marjorie's greatest achievement." Now, years later, Nate agreed and knew the reason why. She was sleeping with her head on his chest.

Nate and Sharon never talked about their legacy and living a life well lived with other people. They both agreed that it might sound like bragging. Such talk should be left for others to share. They did enjoy sharing their thoughts on the subject with each other. Nate and Sharon had so many years of stories of good deeds and positive support to reminisce about. The couple also knew the value, the love, the kindness, and the words they had for each other for all these years were so, so, very special. Their marriage, full of joy and happiness, contributed significantly to them giving so much to so many.

Epilogue

The JT Ranch was given to the state as a historical park in 1955. Ruthie and Sammy's daughter, Sharon M, was head of the JT Ranch Foundation. She had explained to the family that the JT would have to be updated to a large degree if it was to continue being a viable hotel and dude ranch. The family favored keeping everything the same. They liked the idea of people coming to see the history and legacy of this one of a kind ranch. The family wanted the public to see the JT House; it was registered as a historical building. Riding in the old work wagons might be fun for many. People fond of American history might enjoy the two sawmills, blacksmithing and wood shop areas, and the water system. They all still worked, but the work areas hadn't been used in a number of years. The board agreed to give it to the state.

Ruthie had spearheaded the development of the JT Ranch Foundation in 1950. There was a rather large amount of money to be managed and nobody nearby to make all the big decisions, except for Ruthie, Sammy, and Sharon M. Lizzie, Steve, and their whole family lived on the western slopes of the Sierra Nevada Mts. in California. Sally, Susan, and all their kin had moved to Colorado. Andy and Bethany were in Florida near where their daughter lived. Henry, Donald, and their wives were in Chicago. Ruthie got a unanimous agreement that there would be one board member from each of the girls' families; the Browns and Andy's family would also have one each. Sammy was also on the board, thus giving his family two votes. Everyone in the family agreed that since Ruthie and Sammy were on the ranch, it would be appropriate for their family to have two votes. The two other board members came from the town, elected by the seven Johnson clan members.

Sharon M. Johnson was the only board member who was paid a full salary in 1955. The CEO was on the premises just about every day. She was actively involved with the state and all the employees, coordinating and organizing everything in regards to the JT Ranch.

The Johnson family wanted the public to have access to the entire area of the ranch from May 1 thru the month of October, but it was still functioning as a ranch throughout the year. There were still horse rentals, a small herd of cattle, and a lovely garden. The orchard was as beautiful as ever. Jam was still being made. All these things needed someone's attention. The state liked that someone was taking care of the ranch when the park was officially closed. Ruthie had told the entire Johnson clan years earlier that her daughter had the strongest connection to the JT that she had ever seen. Sharon M. was always happiest when she was at the ranch; the future CEO especially liked Legacy Park.

On the weekends during the park's open season, the parking lot near the entrance was usually full with an overflow of cars parking on the streets nearby. The state hired all the personnel who worked at the ranch. There were eight full-time employees and several part- time workers. Ruthie's family lived nearby and worked on the ranch. Ruthie and Sammy didn't work a full week. They mostly supervised and provided much enjoyment to anyone they might come across. They still loved horses and working in the garden together. Their daughter had seen the same behavior some years earlier when she was a small child.

Sammy had done a thorough job of getting volunteers to work in the woodworking shop. The men and a few women worked and answered questions from the visitors in the area. The "crew" made little items that were sold in the gift shop at the SAMM House. People seemed to love watching the volunteers work; it really seemed to help sales. The lumber mills were on display with a docent in each area, but the Board decided they were not to function. The noise the mills created ruined the tranquility of the area. The same was true for the blacksmithing area.

Ruthie and Sharon M had lined up quite a few docents to work at the Park. The whole town loved the JT Ranch. Sammy and Ruthie were often seen walking around near the horses and the shops. They loved talking about the history of the JT. They always made it a point to visit with any docents they might come across. The couple issued many heartfelt thank you, smiles, and compliments to the volunteers.

The JT Ranch Foundation benefitted the ranch and the town. The Johnson family had never stopped supporting the town; it was part of their legacy. The Foundation was the idea of Doris and Mac's son. There was so much money in the bank. Mac Jones Jr. and a few friends had been very successful in managing their money. They lent their expertise to the Foundation for a little while to help get things started. It didn't take long for the JT Ranch Foundation to be quite a successful operation. Mac Jr. didn't want to be on the board. He and his friends decided it would be best if they just continued to advise the Board on financial matters. All of them loved the ranch. They took their job advising the Foundation very seriously. Mac Jr. had taught his friends about the power of giving. The group always donated a rather large amount of money every year to maintain one of their favorite places.

Ruthie and then Sharon M. had been the only two CEOs of the Foundation. They both completely loved the work. The rest of the board members received small stipends. The Foundation was constantly in touch with the town. It was always there to support children activities and any town projects; children activities were always the priority. Each year the Foundation awarded two scholarships, THE NATE and THE SHARON. They were very prestigious.

Nate and Sharon had left a substantial amount of money to the family to ensure the care of the ranch, especially Legacy Park. It was such a special place. The largest amount of money in the Foundation's coffers was the money from Dan Perkins and Colonel Jones' estates. There was so much land; no one knew that they had purchased another 10,000 acres of timberland right next to their original 10,000. The mill had been immediately successful, and there was so much money coming in that the two owners didn't know what to do with it. The Colonel suggested they purchase more land; Dan agreed. In addition, Dan is old mine property that he had bought when he first came to town was now very close to the train depot. It had also become quite valuable.

There were many things to do at the historical park. People could hike in the hills or walk the grounds. Volunteers from the town had built two trails through the park; they also maintained them. The visitors could take a wagon ride out to Dan and Rich's sawmill operation or over to the Small Ranch. They were both part of the park. There were four old ranch wagons operating. A visitor bought a pass and rode whenever it fit their schedule. People really liked that. Legacy Park was the place where everybody spent significant time reading and looking around. These visits frequently generated sales in the gift shop.

Horseback riding over to the Small Ranch or out past the Jones-Perkins Mill were popular. The entire area had always been quite beautiful. It was now even better, especially in late spring. Sharon and her girls had planted so many trees. The new growth in the spring, the birds and squirrels, and just the aesthetics of the area thrilled the riders and the hikers. One more item that Nate and Sharon left behind were wildflowers and some other types with pretty blooms that did well in the area. The couple had spread them around different areas of the two ranches. They were stunning during the first three months of the park's opening. .

The park remained popular for many years. One rather notable piece of information was that not virtually all the people working as paid employees, volunteers, or docents at the park leaved. Most of them felt that this place was special. Many good things were happening here. The entire crew enjoyed the visitors. The conversations were almost always very pleasant in nature. People seemed to smile so much while at the park.

While Sharon M. was the CEO, she noticed something interesting. There seemed to be an influx of money into the foundation from strangers. The number of donations from strangers seemed to be increasing every year. Most of the Johnson clan gave contributions on a yearly basis. Sharon always wrote a little note to personalize the thank you to the family. She always kept a record of all donations and always sent thank you on the official Foundation letterhead. She actually had to get some help to keep up with all the work. Luckily, she had a couple of friends who were more than willing to help.

It didn't take long before the three women knew why so many strangers were contributing to the Foundation. Many of the enclosed letters stated that this beautiful park needed to be preserved. They mentioned the history, the splendid old buildings and work areas, and the grounds that were all so very special. The visitors explained that they had read everything at Legacy Park. Those wonderful words had quite an effect on them. They were so impressed that when they went to the gift shop to look around, they bought some of the pamphlets. The pamphlets were simply amazing. The visitors showed them to family and friends; the pamphlets changed lives. The one book, **Nate and Sharon,** also sold very well. IT WAS SO VERY SPECIAL

Doris and her son, Mac Jr., wrote the book together. Mac Jr. had combined his dad's love of history and his mother's knack for writing. He had published seven books prior to this one. This tribute to his uncle and aunt, according to many, was his best. He and his mom believed it was a story that had to be told, but only after the amazing couple had taken their perch overlooking their "flock".

Sharon and her friends knew the power of Legacy Park; they were frequent visitors. They would always go their separate ways when they got to the park. It was a time for reflection. Sharon didn't know what her friends did, but she read the headstones of the upper two tiers every time she visited. She thanked the mentors for their lessons. Each visit for Sharon was rejuvenating. She was so proud that her last name was Johnson.

One day after spending some time at the park, Sharon's friend, Janice, said that it appears that the mentors on the two upper tiers are still performing quite well. Can you believe it? The words in the park, along with Doris' pamphlets and the Jones' book, are still teaching lessons to so many. These wonderful life lessons are being passed from person to person, family to family, and even from generation to generation. There are so many great lessons,

ALL CONTRIBUTING TO SO MANY LIVES WELL LIVED.

There's Always Questions.

Reviewing what we have read enhances learning. Discuss and/or complete a writing assignment for the following questions.

1. Explain the following lessons along with your thoughts.

A. compliments B. smiles C. framework of a house D. small talk E. giving to others F. being kind – showing respect G. gossip and bullying H. everyone a flower

I. oral communication J. work ethic K. unspoken communication

1. Nate really liked his mother's lesson on how to learn to work together in the garden and with the animals. Your thoughts
2. Mention at least four things Nate did for Sharon – one point for each. Name six more to score a ten.
3. Sitting on the porch at the JT became something special for Nate and Sharon. Why?

   Your thoughts

4. How did Sharon's life before Nate prepare her for him? How did Nate's first twenty-one years prepare him for Sharon?
5. Sharon was kind to all people for several reasons. Your thoughts
6. Thomas' idea of having Nate teach Marjorie was great. How did it prepare him for things to come?
7. The first day Nate and Sharon worked together while Thomas went for lumber was rather special. Explain.
8. Please comment on why Mary was so special. Answer should be about one page.
9. The family thought mentoring was a very special thing. Your thoughts
10. Write a two-page piece on the reflection of his life that went through Thomas' mind when he was 69 years old.

11. Can you imagine how Nate and Sharon Moore felt after visiting the JT Ranch and the
12. Small Ranch as young adults? Your thoughts
13. Mac Jr. and Doris wrote quite a tribute about Nate and Sharon. Write a two page original piece highlighting five major parts of the book.
14. Nate and Sharon created many mentors. Write a two page original story about one or two of these mentors. Include lessons that might have been passed on.
15. Create a two page original story about Sharon befriending a young mother. Use Ruthie and Lizzie as assistants. Sharon had babysat for money per her dad's orders. She really enjoyed the activity. The story should contain a number of Sharon's "learned skills".
16. Nate told Sharon that, in his opinion, she had surpassed M's accomplishments. Explain why he felt this way.
17. Nate was Marjorie and Thomas' greatest achievement. Explain.
18. Nate learned to "Do no harm" with his words or actions. He never forgot this. Instead, he focused on kindness and respect. In today's world, many do not always seem to practice Nate's lessons on "Do no harm". Your thoughts
19. After reading the book, a person might understand more about good mentoring and appreciate its effects. Create a story that demonstrates good mentoring.
20. The Moore family bought a beautiful horse ranch. Tom and Michelle knew the previous owners, Dottie and Hank Toledo. They were the owners of the business where Tom was employed. Dottie and Hank wanted the Moores to buy the ranch. The Moores had visited the ranch often, and every Moore loved everything about the ranch. After the purchase, Nate and Sharon Moore and their families actually lived on the ranch. All the Moores were close by. Write a story about the family interaction at the ranch using some of Nate and Sharon's lessons.

Many more topics could be discussed and/or written about. Be creative, original, and enjoy the "journey".

Made in the USA
Columbia, SC
17 April 2025

1725be1b-a3a6-48b2-bf79-6ca0ce23ab70R01